Lecture Notes in Computer Science　　10549

Commenced Publication in 1973
Founding and Former Series Editors:
Gerhard Goos, Juris Hartmanis, and Jan van Leeuwen

More information about this series at http://www.springer.com/series/7412

M. Jorge Cardoso · Tal Arbel et al. (Eds.)

Imaging for Patient-Customized Simulations and Systems for Point-of-Care Ultrasound

International Workshops, BIVPCS 2017 and POCUS 2017
Held in Conjunction with MICCAI 2017
Québec City, QC, Canada, September 14, 2017
Proceedings

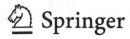 Springer

Editors
M. Jorge Cardoso
University College London
London
UK

Tal Arbel
McGill University
Montreal, QC
Canada

Workshop Editors *see next page*

ISSN 0302-9743   ISSN 1611-3349 (electronic)
Lecture Notes in Computer Science
ISBN 978-3-319-67551-0   ISBN 978-3-319-67552-7 (eBook)
DOI 10.1007/978-3-319-67552-7

Library of Congress Control Number: 2017953408

LNCS Sublibrary: SL6 – Image Processing, Computer Vision, Pattern Recognition, and Graphics

Printed on acid-free paper

This Springer imprint is published by Springer Nature
The registered company is Springer International Publishing AG
The registered company address is: Gewerbestrasse 11, 6330 Cham, Switzerland

Workshop Editors

International Workshop on Bio-Imaging and Visualization for Patient-Customized Simulations, BIVPCS 2017

João Manuel R.S. Tavares ⓘ
Universidade do Porto
Porto
Portugal

Shuo Li ⓘ
University of Western Ontario
London, ON
Canada

International Workshop on Point-of-Care Ultrasound: Algorithms, Hardware, and Applications, POCUS 2017

Stephen Aylward
Kitware Inc.
Carrboro, NC
USA

Luv Kohli
InnerOptic Technology
Hillsborough, NC
USA

Emad Boctor
Johns Hopkins University
Baltimore, MD
USA

Deborah Shipley Kane
Washington University Medical Center
St. Louis, MO
USA

Gabor Fichtinger
Queen's University
Kingston, ON
Canada

Matt Oetgen
Children's National Medical Center
Washington, DC
USA

Kevin Cleary
Children's National Medical Center
Washington, DC
USA

Sonja Pujol
Brigham and Women's Hospital
Boston, MA
USA

Bradley Freeman
Washington University Medical Center
St. Louis, MO
USA

International Workshop on Bio-Imaging and Visualization for Patient-Customized Simulations, BIVPCS 2017

Imaging and Visualization are among the most dynamic and innovative areas of research of the past few decades. Justification of this activity arises from the requirements of important practical applications such as the visualization of computational data, the processing of medical images for assisting medical diagnosis and intervention, and the 3D geometry reconstruction and processing for computer simulations.

Currently, due to the development of more powerful hardware resources and mathematical and physical methods, researchers have been incorporating advanced computational techniques to derive sophisticated methodologies that can better solve the problems encountered. Consequently, effective methodologies have been proposed, validated, and in some cases integrated into commercial software for computer simulations.

The main goal of this MICCAI workshop on Bio-Imaging and Visualization for Patient-Customized Simulations is to provide a platform for communication among specialists from complementary fields such as signal and image processing, mechanics, computational vision, mathematics, physics, informatics, computer graphics, bio-medical practice, psychology, and industry. Another important objective of this MICCAI workshop is to establish a viable connection between software developers, specialist researchers, and applied end-users from diverse fields related to signal processing, imaging, visualization, biomechanics, and simulation.

This book contains the full papers presented at the MICCAI 2017 workshop on Bio-Imaging and Visualization for Patient-Customized Simulations (BIVPCS 2017), which was organized under the auspices of the 20th International Conference on Medical Image Computing and Computer Assisted Intervention 2017, held in Quebec City, Quebec, Canada, during September 10–14, 2017. BIVPCS 2017 brought together researchers representing several fields, such as biomechanics, engineering, medicine, mathematics, physics, and statistics. The works included in this book present and discuss new trends in those fields, using several methods and techniques, including the finite element method, muscle mechanics, computational fluid dynamics, convolutional neural networks, similarity metrics, histograms of oriented gradients, local binary pattern descriptors, non-negative matrix factorization, local cumulative spectral histograms, partial least squares regression, atlas, level-set thresholding, k-means clustering, deformable models, and sensors calibration, in order to address more efficiently different and timely applications involving signal and image acquisition, image processing and analysis, image segmentation, image classification, image reconstruction, image registration, 2D-3D reconstruction, computer simulation, image based modelling, image based diagnosis, surgery planning and simulation, and therapy planning.

The editors wish to thank all the BIVPCS 2017 authors and members of the Program Committee for sharing their expertise, and also the MICCAI Society for having hosted and supported the workshop within MICCAI 2017.

September 2017   João Manuel R.S. Tavares
                                                                                    Shuo Li

Organization

Organizing Committee

João Manuel R.S. Tavares   Faculdade de Engenharia da Universidade do Porto, Porto, Portugal

Shuo Li   University of Western Ontario, London, Canada

Program Committee

Chunming Li	University of Electronic Science and Technology, China
Daniela Lacoviello	Università degli Studi di Roma "La Sapienza", Italy
Da-Chuan Cheng	China Medical University, Taiwan
Eduardo Soudah	International Center for Numerical Methods · in Engineering, Spain
Fatima L.S. Nunes	Universidade de São Paulo, Brazil
Fiorella Sgallari	University of Bologna, Italy
Guoyan Zheng	University of Bern, Switzerland
Hu Zhenghui	Zhejiang University of Technology, China
James S. Duncan	Yale University, USA
João Paulo Papa	Universidade Estadual Paulista, Brazil
Khan M. Iftekharuddin	Old Dominion University, USA
Leo Joskowicz	The Hebrew University of Jerusalem, Israel
Liansheng Wang	Xiamen University, China
Manuel González Hidalgo	Balearic Islands University, Spain
Michel Audette	Old Dominion University, USA
Miguel Velhote Correia	Universidade do Porto, Portugal
Nishikant Deshmukh	Johns Hopkins University, USA
Paola Lecca	University of Trento, Italy
Paolo Emilio Puddu	Sapienza University of Rome, Italy
Prahlad G. Menon	University of Pittsburgh, USA
Reneta Barneva	State University of New York Fredonia, USA
Sanderson L. Gonzaga de Oliveira	Universidade Federal de Lavras, Brazil
Sidney Fels	University of British Columbia, Canada
Xiuquan Du	Anhui University, China
Yongjie Zhang	Carnegie Mellon University, USA
Yuanjie Zheng	Shandong Normal University, China

Yunliang Cai   Worcester Polytechnic Institute, USA
Zeyun Yu   University of Wisconsin at Milwaukee, USA
Zhen Ma   Universidade do Porto, Portugal
Zhiyun Xue   National Institutes of Health, USA
Ziyue Xu   National Institutes of Health, USA

International Workshop on Point-of-Care Ultrasound, POCUS 2017

Point-of-Care Ultrasound (POCUS) encompasses automated ultrasound image and RF data analysis algorithms, rugged ultrasound probes, robust tracking hardware, and specialized user interfaces including augmented reality systems. The goal of a POCUS system is to guide novice users to properly manipulate a ultrasound probe and interpret the acquired data. The output of a POCUS system is typically a quantitative measure or an automated diagnosis, not a B-mode image. POCUS applications range from detecting intra-abdominal bleeding at the scene of an accident to in-home monitoring of liver health. The POCUS workshop featured invited and accepted presentations, live demonstrations, and a panel discussion.

September 2017

Stephen Aylward
Emad Boctor
Gabor Fichtinger
Kevin Cleary
Matt Oetgen
Deborah Kane
Bradley Freeman
Luv Kohli
Sonia Pujol

Organization

Organizing Committee

Stephen Aylward   Kitware, USA
Emad Boctor   Johns Hopkins University, USA
Gabor Fichtinger   Queens University, Canada
Kevin Cleary   Children's National Medical Center, USA
Matt Oetgen   Children's National Medical Center, USA
Deborah Kane   Washington University, USA
Bradley Freeman   Washington University, USA
Luv Kohli   InnerOptic, USA
Sonia Pujol   Brigham and Women's Hospital, USA

Contents

**International Workshop on Point-of-Care Ultrasound:
Algorithms, Hardware, and Applications, POCUS 2017**

International Workshop on Bio-Imaging and Visualization for Patient-Customized Simulations, BIVPCS 2017

Cortical Envelope Modeling for Interactive Patient-Customized Curvilinear Reformatting in the Native Space

Wallace Souza Loos[1,3](✉), Clarissa Lin Yasuda[2,3](✉), Fernando Cendes[2,3](✉), and Shin-Ting Wu[1,3](✉)

[1] School of Electrical and Computer Engineering, Campinas, Brazil
cmp.wallace@gmail.com, ting@dca.fee.unicamp.br
[2] School of Medical Sciences, Campinas, Brazil
cyasuda2807@gmail.com, fcendes@gmail.com
[3] BRAINN Research, Innovation and Dissemination Center,
University of Campinas, Campinas, Brazil

Abstract. Focal cortical dysplasia is one of the most common cause of medically refractory epilepsy. Its imaging features include cortical architectural abnormalities and abnormal structural arrangement at the interface between the grey matter and the white matter. It is well-known that curvilinear multiplanar reformatting (CMPR), consisting in re-slicing the brain almost prependicular to the inward folding gyri from the view of anatomical planes, enhances the visualization of these abnormalities. In this paper, we present yet another interactive modeling of a patient-customized cortical envelope with which we can automatically re-slice the brain volume in a fashion similar to CMPR. Although our proposal requires fewer user interactions in comparison with the previous proposals, we show that the outcomes of re-slicing match those of the conceived CMPR.

1 Introduction

According to the World Health Organization, approximately 50 million people around the world have epilepsy, making it one of the most common neurological diseases globally [14]. Focal cortical dysplasia (FCD) is a malformation of cortical development (MCD), which is one of the most common cause of medically refractory epilepsy [6]. In the majority of FCD cases the findings on magnetic resonance imaging (MRI) scan are: cortical thickening or thinning, blurring of the grey–white junction, brain atrophy, and hyperintense signals in the grey and subcortical white matter, sometimes with tapering toward the ventricle [8]. Some of these features, such as cortical thickening and the grey matter–white matter transition, cannot be appropriately assessed with multiplanar reformatting because of possible oblique slicing of the cerebral cortex.

For addressing this problem, Bastos *et al.* [1] proposed curvilinear multiplanar reformatting (CMPR) to enhance the display of the grey–white matter

M.J. Cardoso et al. (Eds.): BIVPCS/POCUS 2017, LNCS 10549, pp. 3–10, 2017.
DOI: 10.1007/978-3-319-67552-7_1

transition areas where 74% of patients with FCD present some abnormalities [7]. It consists of peeling off the layers of the brain, like peeling layers of an onion, such that the complex cerebral cortical structures are cut, from the view of anatomical planes, along an approximately perpendicular orientation in relation to the inward folding gyri. The red solid line in Fig. 1(a) illustrates their idea. To put this idea into practice, Bastos *et al.* further proposed manual delineation of the guide curves at several user-selected 2D images. Then, piecewise linear interpolations are applied to build a grid mesh that fits the input data. This mesh represents the cortical envelope that will be used to reformat the data volume. To improve the smoothness of the user-delineated contour, Wansapura *et al.* [13] proposed to interpolate the input data with splines. A problem with the guide curve procedures is that it demands much time for routine clinical use. In Sect. 2 we show that our proposed procedure can model the cortical envelope with many fewer user interactions.

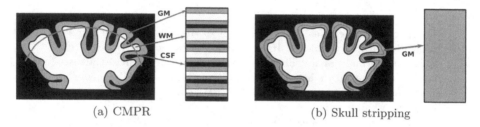

(a) CMPR   (b) Skull stripping

Fig. 1. The curvilinear slicing geometry, in red, originally conceived to CMPR (a) and reached with a skull stripping-based algorithm (b). (Color figure online)

Departing from the mesh approach, Bergo and Falcão [2] proposed to implement CMPR on top of image processing foundations. They apply the Image Forest Transform (IFT) technique to segment the cortical envelope and the Euclidean distance transform of the cortical envelope to control the slicing depth. Huppertz *et al.* [4] proposed to employ a set of predefined standard masks for removing the skull and the brain tissue, step by step, in layers of 2-mm thickness parallel to the outermost mask on the brain surface. They suggest to normalize the source image with the use of the algorithm of the Statistical Parametric Mapping (SPM2). Although not clearly stated in the references of the latest version of BrainSight® [10], we conjecture that it has evolved to the direction of skull stripping followed by automatic reformatting of the brain in 3D curvilinear slices. At interactive rates, the skull is fully removed in the native space, i.e. in the patient-centered reference system, and the remaining brain is automatically sliced parallel to the uncovered surface inwards.

Our concern is that the main goal of non-brain removal algorithms [5,12,17] is to extract the voxels occupied by the brain tissue whose outer layer (cerebral cortex) is not smooth, as shows the red solid line in Fig. 1(b). Note that parallel curves to this red solid line cannot expose the grey–white matter transition so well as that in Fig. 1(a). Because no precise details with respect to the brain's envelope shape are provided by the mask-based CMPR techniques, it is hard to assess how close they approach the original idea. In addition, the non-brain fiducial anatomic landmarks are removed in these techniques. Our proposal not only preserves the fiducial landmarks as illustrates in Figs. 5 and 6, but also provides an almost orthogonal slicing for all cerebral sulci and gyri.

Back to the mesh approach, Wu *et al.* [16] proposed an interactive way to make the CMPR in the native space. Instead of a mask-based approach to remove the skull, the user selects a region on the scalp. This region is sampled and a mesh is created. The mesh is then displaced along the inverse mesh normal direction at the point where the vertex is located. There are, nevertheless, some flaws with this method. It is based on the visibility algorithm and a single view cannot cover the entire cerebral cortex for comparative investigations of the brain. Another problem is the usage of the scalp's geometry as the reference for parallel curvilinear slicing. This may lead to undesirable oblique brain cutting because of differences in the shape of the scalp and that of the cortical envelope. In Sect. 2.2 we present a novel way to construct the re-slicing mesh that approaches the cortical envelope and covers both the right and left hemispheres.

The contributions of our work can be summarized in: (1) the way that we model and adhere the cortical envelope to the dura-mater and (2) the way that the slicing meshes are constructed.

2   Interactive Cortical Envelope Modeling

Our proposal is based on the fact that the dura-mater is a membrane that envelops the brain, and on our finding that the signals of dura-mater are sligtly brighter than the skull and the cerebrospinal fluid (CSF) on a 3.0-T T1-weighted magnetic resonance (T1wMR) scan. We infer that a triangular mesh approximating these detectable brighter signals should be able to re-slice the brain in a CMPR fashion. Hence, we devise a two-step interactive cortical envelope modeling: pre-processing of T1wMR volumes to enhance the transition from the dark skull and the subtly brighter dura-mater, and building a triangular mesh of the cortical envelope on the basis of this transition.

2.1   Suppressing Details

Though not visually perceptible, the intensity values may oscillate largely between the scalp and the dura-mater. Figure 2(b) illustrates the intensity variations of the signals we traced along an inward shooting ray from the scalp in Fig. 2(a). To suppress the signals of diverse micro-structures and to make these variations smoother as depicts Fig. 2(d), we blur a T1wMR volume with a Gaussian filter of the size 9 voxels $\times$ 9 voxels $\times$ 9 voxels ($\sigma = 2$) (Fig. 2(c)). Experimentally, we observed that, despite individual variability, the majority of smoothed signals present the same variation pattern with a local minimum in the skull vault. It is, for example, between the scalp (about 10 mm) and the

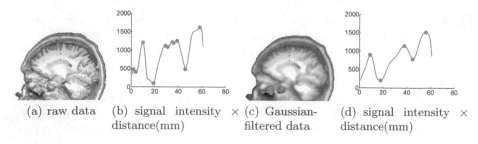

(a) raw data   (b) signal intensity ×   (c) Gaussian-   (d) signal intensity ×
                distance(mm)   filtered data   distance(mm)

Fig. 2. The signal intensity with respect to the distance from the scalp in (a–b) an original T1wMR volume, and (c–d) Gaussian-filtered T1wMR volume.

dura-mater (about 23 mm) in Fig. 2(d). We associated this local minimum to the transition between the skull and the dura-mater. To avoid overlooking this local minimum when we trace the shooting ray at discrete steps, we adopt as the step size the minimum of the half of the voxel dimensions.

2.2   Cortical Envelope

Since the dura-mater's brighter signals are often not continuous due to the T1wMR sampling resolution, improving the transition signals from the dark skull and subtly brighter dura-mater is not enough for segmenting the dura-mater. Inspired by the works of Bastos et al. [1] and Wu et al. [16], we propose to deform a sphere triangular mesh toward the detectable brighter signals corresponding to dura-mater for reconstructing the most likely cortical envelope. The procedure comprises five steps (Fig. 3): (1) interactive removal of background noise with the use of an enhanced threshold filter described in [15] (Fig. 3(a)); (2) automatic placement of the center of a sphere mesh, with the radius equal to 55% of the largest dimension of the volume, at $\overline{C} = \frac{\sum_{i=1}^{n} P_i}{n}$, where P_i are position coordinates of all n valid voxels (Fig. 3(b)); (3) interactive configuration of the region of interest through a clipping plane and of the maximal search depth D for the dura-mater (Fig. 3(c)); (4) automatic deformation of the sphere mesh into a scalp envelop (Fig. 3(d)); and (5) automatic deformation of the scalp

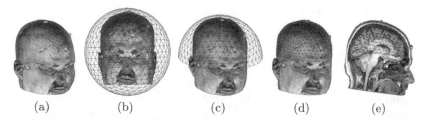

(a)   (b)   (c)   (d)   (e)

Fig. 3. Cortical envelope modeling pipeline: (a) filtered data, (b) sphere mesh, (c) initial deforming mesh, (d) scalp envelope, and (e) cortical envelope.

envelop into the cortical envelop by moving the vertices of scalp envelop toward the brighter signals of dura-mater not greater than D (Fig. 3(e)).

3   Slicing Mesh Quality

Because of its curvilinear shape, the parallel slicing meshes present different triangle sizes and different curvatures at each vertex while we move the cortical envelope inwards. A trial-and-error approach has been conducted for assessing the resolution of the cortical envelope that may prevent degenerate triangles and self-intersection. Three exhaustive experiments have been performed. First, we measured for a slicing mesh with N triangles at the distance d from the cortical envelope its quality $Q_d = \frac{\sum_{t=1}^{N} \lambda(t)}{N}$, where $\lambda(t) = \frac{4\sqrt{3}w(t)}{l_1^2(t)+l_2^2(t)+l_3^2(t)}$ is a measure of triangle compactness in function of its area $w(t)$ and the lengths $l_i(t)$ of its edges [3]. Figure 4(a) is the plot $Q_d \times d$ of the sequence of slicing meshes. The initial mesh of this plot at $0\,\mathrm{mm}$ contains around $N = 640$ triangles. Then, it is displaced at the depth of $40\,\mathrm{mm}$.

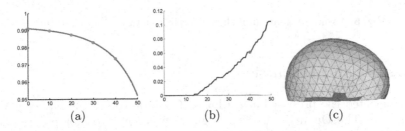

(a)   (b)   (c)

Fig. 4. Numerical evaluations of the quality and the degeneracy of the slicing mesh: (a) quality × distance (mm), (b) degeneracy × distance (mm) and (c) degenerated triangles.

Second, we measured the mesh degeneracy from the ratio R_d of the number of triangles, that tend to shrink to a point, relative to the total number N of triangles in the slicing mesh $\mathcal{M}$ at the distance d. For each displacement Δd, an adaptive threshold is computed and every triangle with the area lower than it is labeled as degenerate. Empirically, we set as the threshold 28% of the largest triangle area of the mesh. Figure 4(b) presents the curve of $R_d \times d$ for an initial mesh with $N = 640$ triangles. Note in Fig. 4(b) that about 6% of the total triangles of the mesh, more precisely 39 triangles, are labeled as degenerate at the depth of $40\,\mathrm{mm}$, as illustrated. A careful analysis shows us that all degenerate triangles are on the border of the deforming mesh. Therefore, they will not affect the slicing quality. Figure 4(c) shows the location of the degenerate triangles, in red, from the left side view of a mesh at the depth of $40\,\mathrm{mm}$.

Finally, we evaluated the visual cropping quality with meshes of different resolution. Figure 5 shows a brain cropped by a slicing mesh of 200, 640 and

2,634 triangles. Visually it is imperceptible the difference between the CMPR slices obtained with 640 triangles (Fig. 5(b)) and the CMPR slices which utilized meshes of higher resolution (Fig. 5(c)), whereas the mesh with 200 triangles cannot fit the cortical envelope well (Fig. 5(a)). To trade-off performance and slicing quality, we decided for an initial tessellated sphere of 1,280 triangles in our implementation and no degeneracy checking was performed along the mesh deformation.

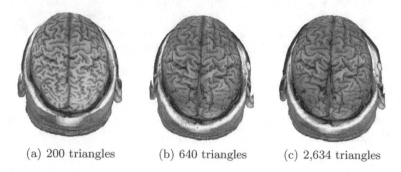

(a) 200 triangles   (b) 640 triangles   (c) 2,634 triangles

Fig. 5. Visual evaluation of slicing quality at the depth ≈20 mm.

4   Results and Discussion

We implemented the proposed algorithm in C++ on top of the half-edge data structure [9]. The OpenGL shading language was employed for programming the graphics processing unit (GPU) [11][1] to improve the performance of our proposed algorithm. On a *desktop* Intel ®Core i7 2.8 GHz with 8 GB of RAM and graphic card NVIDIA GTX 650Ti with 1 GB of VRAM spends our algorithm less than 2 s to curvilinearly reformat a volume of dimensions $356 \times 512 \times 512$. All T1wMR test images were acquired with the Philips Achieva 3 T at the hospital of the University of Campinas. The dimensions of most tested MR volumes are either $180 \times 240 \times 240$ or $356 \times 512 \times 512$. All patients enrolled in the present study signed an informed consent form approved by the Ethics Committee of our university.

Figure 6 illustrates results we achieved concerning the quality of our proposal in curvilinearly slicing the brain in the direction that is almost orthogonal to inward folding gyri. We present six different volumes from different view planes. Observe that the green curve, which is the intersection of the T1wMR volume and our proposed slicing mesh, satisfies the CMPR requirement in all cerebral regions except in the temporal pole (Fig. 6(a)). This is because of anatomical connections between the brain and the eyes through the optic chiasm. The intensity variations along the path connecting the scalp and the brain in this region

---

[1] Supplementary video demonstrating curvilinear reformatting on MR-T1 volumes was uploaded as part of this submission.

does not follow the pattern shown in Fig. 2(d). Further studies are necessary to improve the characterization of intensity variations between the scalp and the brain in this region. Note that our proposal also works for non-spherical shaped cortical envelopes, as illustrate Figs. 6(c) and (e).

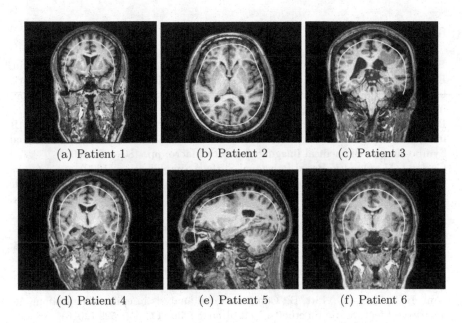

(a) Patient 1   (b) Patient 2   (c) Patient 3

(d) Patient 4   (e) Patient 5   (f) Patient 6

Fig. 6. Slicing a brain in the CMPR fashion. (Color figure online)

Our algorithm requires that the user provides the noise threshold (Fig. 3(a)), the region of the scalp to be curvilinearly reformatted (Fig. 3(c)), and the patient-customized maximal search depth for the dura-mater. Although our algorithm is not fully automatic, the required values are physical measurements that do not involve advanced knowledge about the underlying algorithm and an interactive interface has been designed for accomplishing the three tasks. Usability tests should be performed for assessing its clinical value.

5 Conclusion

We present an interactive CMPR algorithm that distinguishes from previous works in the way that the slicing meshes are constructed. Besides that, the CMPR algorithm presented reformats a brain volume in curvilinear slices parallel to the dura-mater, aiming to better expose the transition area from the gray matter and the white matter. To our best knowledge, it is the first work that provides a deep analysis of the quality of the slicing geometry.

Acknowledgment. The research was supported by a CNPq-Brazil fellowship (305785/2012-5, 308764/2015-3), a CNPq-Brazil scholarship (165777/2014-1), the Fapesp Individual Project grant #2011/02351-0, and the Fapesp-Brazil grant #2013/07559-3 to the BRAINN Research, Innovation and Dissemination Center of the University of Campinas.

References

1. Bastos, A.C., Comeau, R.M., Andermann, F., Melanson, D., Cendes, F., Dubeau, F., Fontaine, S., Tampieri, D., Olivier, A.: Diagnosis of subtle focal dysplastic lesions: curvilinear reformatting from three-dimensional magnetic resonance imaging. Ann. Neurol. **46**(1), 88–94 (1999)
2. Bergo, F.P.G., Falcao, A.: Fast and automatic curvilinear reformatting of MR images of the brain for diagnosis of dysplastic lesions. In: 3rd IEEE International Symposium on Biomedical Imaging: Nano to Macro, pp. 486–489 (2006)
3. Garland, M.: Quadric-Based Polygonal Surface Simplification (1999)
4. Huppertz, H.J., Kassubek, J., Altenmüller, D.M., Breyer, T., Fauser, S.: Automatic curvilinear reformatting of three-dimensional MRI data of the cerebral cortex. NeuroImage **39**(1), 80–86 (2008)
5. Iglesias, J.E., Liu, C.Y., Thompson, P.M., Tu, Z.: Robust brain extraction across datasets and comparison with publicly available methods. IEEE Trans. Med. Imaging **30**(9), 1617–1634 (2011)
6. Kabat, J., Krol, P.: Focal cortical dysplasia - review. Pol. J. Radiol./Pol. Med. Soc. Radiol. **77**(2), 35–43 (2012)
7. Kini, L.G., Gee, J.C., Litt, B.: Computational analysis in epilepsy neuroimaging: a survey of features and methods. NeuroImage Clin. **11**, 515–529 (2016)
8. Leventer, R.J., Guerrini, R., Dobyns, W.B.: Malformations of cortical development and epilepsy. Dialogues Clin. Neurosci. **10**(1), 47–62 (2008)
9. Mäntylä, M.: An Introduction to Solid Modeling. Computer Science Press Inc., New York (1987)
10. Rogue Research, Inc.: BrainSight - User Manual, Version 1.7. Accessed October 2016
11. Sellers, G., Wright, R.S., Haemel, N.: OpenGL Superbible: Comprehensive Tutorial and Reference, 7th edn. Addison-Wesley Professional, Toronto (2015)
12. Smith, S.M.: Fast robust automated brain extraction. Hum. Brain Mapp. **17**(3), 143–155 (2002). http://dx.doi.org/10.1002/hbm.10062
13. Wansapura, J.P., Williams, O.L., Williams, J.M., Mandybur, G.: A Simple Algorithm for Curvilinear Reformatting of 3D MRI Data (2003). http://cds.ismrm.org/ismrm-2003/0892.pdf
14. World Health Organization: World health organization: Epilepsy, October 2016. http://www.who.int/mediacentre/factsheets/fs999/en/
15. Wu, S.T., Valente, A.C., de Souza Watanabe, L., Yasuda, C.L., Coan, A.C., Cendes, F.: Pre-alignment for Co-registration in Native Space. In: 2014 27th SIBGRAPI Conference on Graphics, Patterns and Images, pp. 41–48, August 2014
16. Wu, S.T., Yasuda, C.L., Cendes, F.: Interactive curvilinear reformatting in native space. IEEE Trans. Visual. Comput. Graph. **18**(2), 299–308 (2012)
17. Zhang, H., Liu, J., Zhu, Z., Li, H.: An automated and simple method for brain MR image extraction. BioMed. Eng. OnLine **10**(1), 81 (2011)

Simulation of Patient-Specific Deformable Ultrasound Imaging in Real Time

Mafalda Camara[✉], Erik Mayer, Ara Darzi, and Philip Pratt

Department of Surgery and Cancer, Imperial College, London, UK
m.camara15@imperial.ac.uk

Abstract. Intraoperative ultrasound is an imaging modality frequently used to provide delineation of tissue boundaries. This paper proposes a simulation platform that enables rehearsal of patient-specific deformable ultrasound scanning in real-time, using preoperative CT as the data source. The simulation platform was implemented within the GPU-accelerated NVIDIA FleX position-based dynamics framework. The high-resolution particle model is used to deform both surface and volume meshes. The latter is used to compute the barycentric coordinates of each simulated ultrasound image pixel in the surrounding volume, which is then mapped back to the original undeformed CT volume. To validate the computation of simulated ultrasound images, a kidney phantom with an embedded tumour was CT-scanned in the rest position and at five different levels of probe-induced deformation. Measures of normalised cross-correlation and similarity between features were adopted to compare pairs of simulated and ground truth images. The accurate results demonstrate the potential of this approach for clinical translation.

1 Introduction

Intraoperative imaging has been used for navigation in robotic surgical procedures as a mean to compensate for the limited access, narrowed field of view and lack of tactile feedback. In the context of robot-assisted partial nephrectomy (RAPN), intraoperative ultrasound (US) facilitates delineation of the tumour's borders, potentially improves the tumour dissection and minimises the risk of positive margins. The benefit of using such an imaging modality associated with the challenge of acquiring and understanding the data, has encouraged the development of simulation-based environments. Depending on the specific application of the simulator, different features are desired, from real time performance, use of patient-specific data, a biomechanical model to account for deformation and acoustic imaging features. Regarding the use of patient-specific data, by resorting to the GPU and the use of CT volumes, Reichl et al. [1] achieved realistic US images and acoustic features in real time. The similar principle of using imaging volumes and wave propagation techniques has been adopted by Shams et al. [2] and Salehi et al. [3]. The former results in accurate and realistic modelling of acoustic phenomena while using patient-specific data. However, deformation caused by external forces were not integrated into the simulations. Alternatively,

© Springer International Publishing AG 2017
M.J. Cardoso et al. (Eds.): BIVPCS/POCUS 2017, LNCS 10549, pp. 11–18, 2017.
DOI: 10.1007/978-3-319-67552-7_2

some effort has been focused on compensating for deformation. Pheiffer et al. [4] defined a framework for correcting non-rigid tissue compression induced by the probe in US scanning, to allow for a more accurate volume estimation to be used in image guidance. Flach et al. [5] used a FEM model around the contact areas and the known probe geometry to provide an accurate undeformed 3D volume. Similar work was developed by Goksel et al. [6] to simulate B-mode images of deformable tissue. These techniques depend on the use of a priori known 3D US volumes, commonly unavailable in the context of RAPN. Techniques combining 3D volumes and biomechanical modelling have been adopted to address simultaneously deformation and the use of patient-specific data. Selmi et al. [7] developed a method for realistic 3D deformable US image generation in real time. A biomechanical model was combined with a 3D elastic texture in order to re-slice the patient's volume to achieve deformable US images. Bürger et al. [8] developed an US simulator for medical education based on a convolution ray-tracing approach and a deformable mesh model. Morin et al. [9] simulated US imaging for breast cancer. MRI volumes in combination with a biomechanical model provided the means to simulate realistic US imaging.

The framework adopted in this paper combines the use of a biomechanical model and a 3D preoperative volume to simulate deformable US images interactively. This biomechanical model was previously implemented and validated for a patient-specific surgical simulator, as described in Camara et al. [10]. The focus of the work is not on modelling realistic US images but rather in providing an accurate simulation platform that ultimately provides the user with the opportunity to rehearse scanning with patient-specific data. Additionally, it can act as a validation context for manually-operated 3D tumour acquisition and reconstruction, and to assist further with the automation of intraoperative scanning protocols. The novel aspect in this paper lays on the deformation method implemented for a patient-specific simulation in real time, associated with a straightforward data preparation that enables a facilitated translation into clinical practice.

2   Methods

2.1   Development of a Partial Nephrectomy Phantom

A kidney phantom with embedded tumour was developed in a methodology similar to the one used by Hughes-Hallett [11]. Polyvinyl alcohol (PVA), a polymer that presents similar tensile strength and elasticity to tissue, can be used as a surrogate for soft tissue organs. A 10% PVA by weight concentration solution was used. Regarding mimicking tissue biomechanics, by subjecting the solution to a certain number of freeze-defrost cycles, one can change the material rigidity. A tumour is often stiffer and less elastic when compared to the surrounding renal parenchyma. Therefore, the tumour was subjected to an initial cycle and the overall phantom to an extra cycle to create realistic kidney properties. With respect to CT imaging the phantom, there was a need to clearly differentiate the boundary between tumour and kidney parenchyma. The tumour was enveloped in a thin layer of dense putty, as it presents an increased radiographic attenuation coefficient and allowed the boundary to be identified. A 3D-printed non-diseased kidney was used as the mould for phantom. The tumour mould was a simple spherical mould with diameter of 2.3 cm.

2.2 Experimental Setup

A rig designed in SolidEdge and 3D-printed with polyamide (Materialise), was used to induce deformation. The rig was composed of a platform designed to support the phantom and a movable structure which represents an US probe. Five different levels of deformation were used (total of 14.6 mm), each inducing approximately a 2.5 mm increment. The bottom part of the kidney mould was used to act as boundary conditions. The combination of mould and kidney was placed within the rig and the movable structure varied its position to desired locations for each set of acquired CT scans. CT images were acquired with a GE Innova 4100 scanner. Initially, the entire setup was CT scanned for no applied deformation. It was always assured that the US probe was positioned as if scanning part of the tumour and that the probe was rigidly fixed. This procedure was continued for the different levels of deformation, by moving the probe to the subsequent level of deformation and CT scanning the setup. The entire setup is showed in Fig. 1(a).

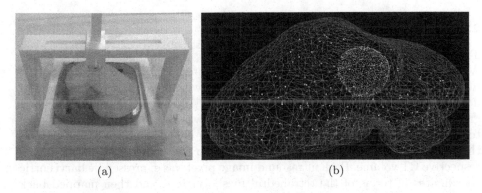

(a)   (b)

Fig. 1. (a) Deformation rig with phantom and support, placed on the CT scanner table. (b) Cluster distribution within tumour (red) and kidney (yellow) meshes. (Color figure online)

2.3 Simulation Platform and Biomechanical Model

The simulation platform was implemented within the GPU-accelerated NVIDIA FleX position-based dynamics framework [12], in a manner similar to that reported in Camara et al. [10]. All structures of interest, i.e. the kidney, tumour, support mesh and structure representing the US probe, were segmented from the 3DCT scans using ITK-SNAP and exported as surface mesh files. Kidney and tumour meshes were imported to MeshLab, whereby smoothed (using the volume-preserving HC Laplacian smoothing algorithm) and decimated (with the quadratic edge collapse decimation algorithm). The FleX framework supports different forms of modelling structure and collision geometries. The tumour mesh was modelled as a triangular mesh, solely used for analysis, whereas the kidney, which embeds the tumour region, was modelled as a combination of particles. These particles were distributed and clustered together into shape-matching clusters, assuming two different values of stiffness coefficients. For all the clusters where centroids were found within the tumour mesh boundaries, the cluster stiffness coefficient modelled the tumour deformation, whereas the remaining clusters were assigned to a different stiffness coefficient to model the kidney deformation. This assured that the approximate regions of kidney and tumour were modelled as different structures. The support structure was represented as a static triangular mesh and used as boundary conditions for the kidney model. The ultrasound transducer (Aloka UST-533) was approximated as a cuboid and modelled as a dynamic convex mesh. Both the vertices of the tumour mesh and triangular mesh representing the kidney surface were defined in accordance with local particle positions through a weighted matrix bending technique, often referred as 'skinning' [13]. Therefore, the structures attached to the particle system deformed in terms of the manipulated kidney parenchyma. The representation of clusters, kidney and tumour surface meshes are showed in Fig. 1(b).

2.4   Ultrasound Simulation

The deformable US scans were simulated by using the same 'skinning' technique. A tetrahedral mesh for the kidney was computed with Gmsh and imported into the simulation. This mesh was embedded within the particle system and deformed in accordance with its displacements. A planar discretisation, i.e. a grid of 1×2 cm with a resolution of $0.25\,\text{mm}$, was registered to the US probe to display the deformable slice, by means of an efficient interpolation method that mapped the simulated ultrasound pixels to the undeformed voxels in the respective CT volume. Each ultrasound image pixel was expressed by barycentric coordinates in terms of the tetrahedral mesh vertices, and then mapped back to the voxels of the respective undeformed CT volume. For each image pixel $\mathbf{p} = [x\ y\ z]^T$, its 3D position within a tetrahedral element t, can be expressed as

$$\mathbf{p} = \sum_{i=0}^{3} \lambda_i \mathbf{r}_i \quad \text{with} \quad \sum_{i=0}^{3} \lambda_i = 1, \lambda_i \geq 0 \tag{1}$$

where λ_i are the barycentric coordinates in terms of the element corners $\mathbf{r}_i = [x_i\ y_i\ z_i]^T$, which represent the deformed 'skinned' vertices. Rearranging Eq. 1 and expressing it in a matrix form, results in

$$\mathbf{T}\boldsymbol{\lambda} = \mathbf{p} - r_3 \tag{2}$$

where the matrix T and the array λ are defined as

$$T = \begin{bmatrix} x_0 - x_3 & x_1 - x_3 & x_2 - x_3 \\ y_0 - y_3 & y_1 - y_3 & y_2 - y_3 \\ z_0 - z_3 & z_1 - z_3 & z_2 - z_3 \end{bmatrix}, \lambda = [\lambda_1 \ \lambda_2 \ \lambda_3]^T$$

The barycentric coordinates can be found solving Eq. 2 for λ,

$$\lambda = T^{-1}(p - r_3) \tag{3}$$

Finally, to recover the pixel texture coordinates from the undeformed voxels, as pixel p is defined by the same barycentric coordinates in the original configuration and the deformed state, one needs to solve the following equation,

$$p = T^0 \lambda + r_3^0 \tag{4}$$

where T^0 and r_i^0 describe the undeformed state and are expressed as

$$T^0 = \begin{bmatrix} x_0^0 - x_3^0 & x_1^0 - x_3^0 & x_2^0 - x_3^0 \\ y_0^0 - y_3^0 & y_1^0 - y_3^0 & y_2^0 - y_3^0 \\ z_0^0 - z_3^0 & z_1^0 - z_3^0 & z_2^0 - z_3^0 \end{bmatrix}, r_i^0 = [x_i^0 \ y_i^0 \ z_i^0]^T$$

To compare the simulated slices with the respective ground truth images, the location of pixels within the grid was registered to the respective CT volume and saved into an image. The process was repeated for all levels of deformation. The mapping technique to estimate both the simulated and ground truth images is similar, but where simulated slices map the grid to the undeformed volume by means of skinning the particle system, the ground truth slices are obtained by mapping the grid to the volume respective of each level of deformation.

2.5   Calibration

An estimation of parameters to model soft tissue deformation of the porcine kidney was achieved in Camara et al. [10], but a calibration is still necessary as the model used here is a phantom presenting different material properties and hence, different deformation behaviour. Therefore, a calibration was performed to determine the framework parameters that allowed for the most realistic deformation modelling and validation of US simulation. A simple two-dimensional search was used to determine the ideal cluster stiffness coefficient of the general kidney parenchyma, for a given particle radius. The stiffness coefficient for clusters embedded within the tumour boundary was defined as 0.95, as the tumour is known to be stiffer than the surrounding kidney parenchyma, for this specific phantom. The particle radius was permitted in the range [2.2, 2.5, 5.7, 3.0, 3.3] mm and the remaining clusters with a stiffness coefficient in a range [0,1]. The simulation sub-steps and sub-steps iterations were defined as 3 and 9, respectively. The metric undergoing minimisation was the difference, in percentage, of the average count of tumour and kidney pixels between the simulated and the ground truth slices.

3   Results

The metric undergoing minimisation achieved a minimum of 4.5%, across all levels of deformation, for a cluster stiffness coefficient of 0.6 and radius of 2.2 mm. The resulting US image for each level of deformation, against the ground truth, is visible in Fig. 2. Normalised cross-correlation and the difference in approximate distances of the upper and lower extends of boundaries between the simulated and ground truth tumour meshes, are showed in Fig. 3. Absolute distance between the same meshes is showed in Fig. 4. For no deformation, these meshes resemble in volume by 97% compared to the 79% achieved for the 5th level of deformation.

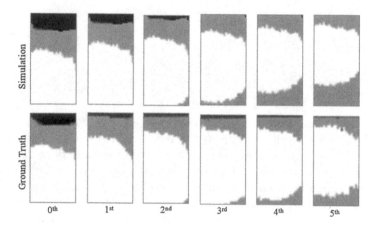

Fig. 2. US images for the increasing levels of deformation (from left to right), of the simulated (top) and ground truth (bottom) slices. Cluster stiffness coefficient was defined as 0.6 and particle radius as 2.2 mm.

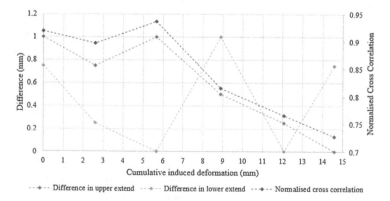

Fig. 3. The left axis represents the difference between the simulated and ground truth slice as a function of the cumulative induced deformation, for the upper and lower extents. The right axis represents the normalised cross-correlation between both images.

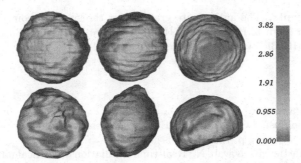

Fig. 4. Representation of the absolute distance (in mm) between the simulated and ground truth tumour meshes. From left to right are represented the anterior, right and inferior views. From top to bottom are represented the 0th and 5th levels of deformation.

4 Discussion and Conclusion

The normalised cross-correlation follows a decreasing trend as the induced deformation increases. The same conclusion is observed in Fig. 2, where the tumour to kidney boundary between the simulated and ground truth images seem to better align for the initial levels of deformation. The tumour meshes in Fig. 4 show similar results, where the pair of meshes presents increasing absolute difference in surface distance for increasing levels of deformation. Regardless of the level of deformation induced by the probe, the difference in the tumour deformation represented in the US slices is smaller than to 1 mm. In the context of an overall displacement of 14.5 mm induced by the US probe, the simulation results in an accurate deformation and visualisation of the US images. The imperfect alignment of the scans and tumour meshes for no applied deformation can only be caused by gravity. Therefore, there is an initial influence on the displacement of particles that was not compensated for throughout the simulation. The use of complex geometries for the phantom and boundary conditions might also influence on the accuracy of the simulation. A three dimensional exhaustive search would have been ideal if accounting for the calibration of the cluster stiffness coefficient for the clusters within the tumour boundaries. Future work will focus on the addition of ultrasound imaging features to improve the realism of the slices. The need for initial gravity compensation will also be addressed. To note that the simulation is patient-specific solely regarding geometry. As described in Miller K. et al. [14], the adoption of patient-specific tissue properties in this family of applications is of secondary importance. Though the simulation uses methodology-based parameters, these can be mapped to real tissue properties in a manner similar to that described in Roberto C. et al. [15].

This paper presents a framework that accurately simulates deformable US slices in real time using patient-specific imaging as source of data. The implemented methodology, which provides a stable and robust real time simulation, coupled with a feasible data preparation, enables a facilitated translation into clinical practice and patient-specific simulation possible on a broader scale.

Acknowledgements. The authors are grateful for the support from the Northwick Park Institute for Medical Research, the Hamlyn Centre for Robotic Surgery and from The Imperial NIHR Biomedical Research Centre (BRC).

References

1. Reichl, T., Passenger, J., Acosta, O., Salvado, O.: Ultrasound goes GPU: real-time simulation using CUDA. In: SPIE Medical Imaging, International Society for Optics and Photonics, p. 726116 (2009)
2. Shams, R., Hartley, R., Navab, N.: Real-time simulation of medical ultrasound from CT images. In: Metaxas, D., Axel, L., Fichtinger, G., Székely, G. (eds.) MICCAI 2008. LNCS, vol. 5242, pp. 734–741. Springer, Heidelberg (2008). doi:10.1007/978-3-540-85990-1_88
3. Salehi, M., Ahmadi, S.-A., Prevost, R., Navab, N., Wein, W.: Patient-specific 3D ultrasound simulation based on convolutional ray-tracing and appearance optimization. In: Navab, N., Hornegger, J., Wells, W.M., Frangi, A.F. (eds.) MICCAI 2015. LNCS, vol. 9350, pp. 510–518. Springer, Cham (2015). doi:10.1007/978-3-319-24571-3_61
4. Pheiffer, T.S., Thompson, R.C., Rucker, D.C., Simpson, A.L., Miga, M.I.: Model-based correction of tissue compression for tracked ultrasound in soft tissue image-guided surgery. Ultrasound Med. Biol. **40**(4), 788–803 (2014)
5. Flack, B., Makhinya, M., Goksel, O.: Model-based compensation of tissue deformation during data acquisition for interpolative ultrasound simulation. In: 2016 IEEE 13th International Symposium Biomedical Imaging (ISBI), pp. 502–505 (2016)
6. Goksel, O., Salcudean, S.E.: B-mode ultrasound image simulation in deformable 3-D medium. IEEE Trans. Med. Imaging **28**(11), 1657–1669 (2009)
7. Selmi, S.-Y., Promayon, E., Sarrazin, J., Troccaz, J.: 3D interactive ultrasound image deformation for realistic prostate biopsy simulation. In: Bello, F., Cotin, S. (eds.) ISBMS 2014. LNCS, vol. 8789, pp. 122–130. Springer, Cham (2014). doi:10.1007/978-3-319-12057-7_14
8. Bürger, B., Bettinghausen, S., Radle, M., Hesser, J.: Real-time GPU-based ultrasound simulation using deformable mesh models. IEEE Trans. Med. Imaging **32**(3), 609–618 (2013)
9. Morin, R., Eiben, B., Bidaut, L., Hipwell, J., Evans, A., Hawkes, D.J.: 3D ultrasound simulation based on a biomechanical model of prone MRI in breast cancer imaging. In: 2015 IEEE 12th International Symposium Biomedical Imaging (ISBI), pp. 264–267 (2015)
10. Camara, M., Mayer, E., Darzi, A., Pratt, P.: Soft tissue deformation for surgical simulation: a position-based dynamics approach. Int. J. Comput. Assist. Radiol. Surg. **11**(6), 919–928 (2016)
11. Hughes-Hallett A.: The image-enhanced operating environment in robot assisted laparoscopic partial nephrectomy. Imperial College London (2016)
12. NVIDIA Gameworks. Nvidia FleX. https://developer.nvidia.com/flex
13. Kavan, L.: Part I: direct skinning methods and deformation primitives. In: ACM SIGGRAPH, pp. 1–11 (2014)
14. Miller, K., Lu, J.: On the prospect of patient-specific biomechanics without patient-specific properties of tissues. J. Mech. Behav. Biomed. Mater. **27**, 154–166 (2013)
15. Rodero, C., Real, P., Zuñeda, P., Monteagudo, C., Lozano, M., García-Fernández, I.: Characterisation of position based dynamics for elastic materials. In: Proceedings of the XXVI Spanish Computer Graphics Conference, pp. 49–57 (2016)

A Hybrid CNN Feature Model for Pulmonary Nodule Differentiation Task

Tingting Zhao[2], Huafeng Wang[1,2(✉)], Lihong Li[3], Yifang Qi[2], Haoqi Gao[2], FangFang Han[4], Zhengrong Liang[5], Yanmin Qi[6], and Yuan Cao[6]

[1] Electrical Information School, North China University of Technology, No. 5, Jinyuanzhuang Road, Shijingshan District, Beijing, China
Wanghuafengbuaa@gmail.com
[2] School of Software, Beihang University, Beijing, China
[3] Department of Engineering Science and Physics, City University of New York at CSI, Staten Island, NY, USA
[4] Department of Biomedical, Northeast University, Shenyan, China
[5] Department of Radiology, State University of New York at Stony Brook, Stony Brook, NY, USA
[6] Civil Aviation Medical Center of Civil Aviation Administration of China, Beijing, China

Abstract. Pulmonary nodule differentiation is one of the most challenge tasks of computer-aided diagnosis(CADx). Both texture method and shape estimation approaches previously presented could provide good performance to some extent in the literature. However, no matter 2D or 3D textures extracted, they just tend to observe characteristics of the pulmonary nodules from a statistical perspective according to local features' change, which hints they are helpless to work as global as the human who always be aware of the characteristics of given target as a combination of local features and global features, thus they have certain limitations. Enlightened by the currently prevailing learning ability of convolutional neural network (CNN) and previously contributions provided by texture features, we here presented a hybrid method for better to complete the differentiation task. It can be observed that our proposed multi-channel CNN model has a better discrimination in capacity according to the projection of distributions of extracted features and achieved a new record with AUC 97.04 on LIDC-IDRI database.

Keywords: Convolutional neural network · Multi-channel CNN · Texture · CADx · Deeplearning · Pulmonary nodule differentiation

1 Introduction

According to statistics from the American Cancer Society, Lung cancer is the first most commonly diagnosed cancer and the first leading cause of death from cancer in the United States, which accounts for 27% of all cancer mortality [6]. Fortunately, early detection and diagnosis of benign or malignancy on those

© Springer International Publishing AG 2017
M.J. Cardoso et al. (Eds.): BIVPCS/POCUS 2017, LNCS 10549, pp. 19–26, 2017.
DOI: 10.1007/978-3-319-67552-7_3

pulmonary nodules can effectively decrease the incidence of lung cancer. Though in the past decades, a large and increasing number of pulmonary nodules have been detected each year by means of the widely using of computer tomography (CT) for lung cancer screening [11], the task of evaluating a large number of detected nodules by the experts or radiologists can still be very burdensome. Therefore, a much better computer-aided diagnosis (CADx) is expected to play an important role in the evaluating task, where the extraction of effective features from detected nodules is of the research interests.

In practice, convolutional neural network (CNN) delivers state-of-the-art performance, which is a derivative of Multilayer Perceptron (MLP) neural networks optimized for two-dimensional pattern recognition. The lack of dependence on prior knowledge and human effort in designing features is a major advantage for CNNs [2,13].

Nevertheless, the feature extraction methods presented by previous artificial designs should still be a useful supplement to CNN features, this paper is to explore the feasibility and validity of the fusion methods among CNN and traditional feature extraction methods by an empirical research. Literately, in 2016, Anirudh R et al. [1] proposed the use of three-dimensional CNN to achieve lung CT image in the nodule location detection, and achieved sensitivities of 80% for 10 false positives per scan. However, to get the 3D labeled training data are really expensive and either are the 3D convolutions; Shen et al. [13] exploited CNN to differentiate lung nodules, and proposed MC-CNN network structure to achieve a 0.93 AUC and 87.14% accuracy on LIDC-IDRI by multi-scale cutting and merging of pooling. As we can see, the classification accuracy and AUC produced by CNN are higher than those of simply produced by traditional methods. Moreover, the result of convolution defines features of input data, such as corners, curves, lines etc. Feature occurrence is mirrored on feature map by corresponding receptive field location, defining features map. After each convolution layer follows subsampling layer. The motivation of this study is to explore a simple way for strengthening the lung nodule feature map by traditional feature incentives, such as HOG and LBP.

As for another challenge of the lung nodule differentiation task be concerned, the original inputs are acquired from CT scans, while in CT scanning, image quality has many components and is influenced by many technical parameters. It is generally considered that the image quality is the main reason why different physicians possibly estimate the same lung nodule with varying reports. So, we argue that if by any other representation of inputs can it bring any gains, such as enhancing the feature of the nodule. In addition, the disadvantage of CNN based methods is that they usually need much large datasets to train a feasible model. Therefore, the main contribution of our new proposed model is to enlarge the training dataset with more feature enhanced inputs given by traditional feature extraction methods and to present a much effective feature model which not only takes advantage of CNN autonomous learned image features, but also the traditional features such as HOG and LBP operators.

2   Method

The overall pipeline of the proposed method is shown in Fig. 1. Firstly, the location of the pulmonary nodule is manually drawn from the lung CT images by up to four radiologists; then all the nodules volumes are extracted automatically from the pulmonary CT images by combining all the radiologists' painting boundaries; next, the hybrid features extracted from the pulmonary volumes will be fed into our proposed CNN models; finally the probability of the benign and malignant be obtained by Softmax classifier.

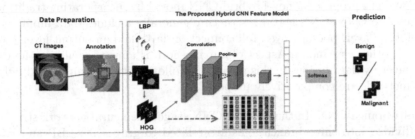

Fig. 1. A schematic diagram of the proposed model

2.1   Histograms of Oriented Gradients (HOG) and Local Binary Pattern (LBP) Descriptors

- HOG: In order to clearly depict the appearance characteristics of lung nodules, Shingo Iwano et al. [14] clinically classified the lung nodules into seven categories: round or oval, lobulated, polygonal, tentacular, spiculated, ragged and other irregular types according to the visual observation from 2D CT images. The idea of HOG stems from the observation that local features such as object appearance and shape can often be characterized well by the distribution of local intensity gradients in the image [4]. HOG features are extracted from an image based on a series of normalized local histograms of image gradient orientations in a dense grid [10]. The HOG feature conveys information that is somewhat like that of an edge map, which also gives the representation some degree of invariance to small and local geometric and photometric changes.
- LBP: Since 1994, LBP has been found to be a powerful feature for texture classification [12]; and it has further been determined that when LBP is combined with the HOG descriptor, it improves the detection performance considerably [15]. Because of the advantage on the powerful illumination invariant, LBP has been widely recognized as a texture operator. This LBP texture operator has been highly successfully used for various computer vision applications, especially for face recognition.

2.2   Hybrid CNN Network Model

Although those previously proposed models such as edge, shape and texture are capable of representing to great certain the characteristic of pulmonary nodules, they are still lack of the ability of generalization and performance varies respectively as far as their designed models to be concerned. By mapping the data into new space through linear or non-linear transformation on the input data, convolutional neural network [2] recently perform very well on the task of extracting the inherent characteristics of the given images. In view of possible complementary characteristics related to traditional texture method and CNN, we thus proposed a novel hybrid CNN model by incorporating traditional features into CNN. CNN network structure generally includes data input layer, convolution layer, pooling layer, full connection layer and an output layer (Softmax and other classifiers). Aspect of our method, it aims to facilitate the data input layer by data fusion. In this paper, the following two feature based hybrid CNN methods are comparatively proposed:

- Multi-branch CNN: In the training CNN stage, the neural network structure is divided into three branches, as are related to gray-scale, LBP and HOG characteristics respectively. Both HOG and LBP features of the lung nodules were extracted as the input of different branches of the CNN and further processed with convolution (as shown in Fig. 2).
- Multi-channel CNN: Although the feature fusion method can effectively exploit the features combined, the fact is that the complexity of the network is increased by 2 times, and the training time is also very consuming. Therefore, a multi-channel feature fusion CNN is proposed. At the beginning of training of CNN, LBP and HOG features are integrated into different channels of the input image, so that local information and global information have been taken into account in training a CNN model (as shown in Fig. 3). Then the input layer changes from $56 \times 56 \times 1$ to $56 \times 56 \times 3$.

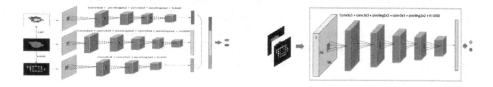

Fig. 2. Multi-branch CNN Model   **Fig. 3.** Multi-channel CNN model

We here describe the cost function that our proposed models used for softmax regression. Given the model parameters θ which were trained to minimize the cost function, and $\theta_1, \theta_2, \ldots, \theta_k \in \mathfrak{R}^{n+1}$ are the parameters of our model. Notice that the term $\sum_{j=1}^{k} e^{\theta_j^T x^{(i)}}$ normalizes the distribution, so that it sums to one. Such that, Softmax regression cost function $J(\theta)$ takes form as,

$$J(\theta) = -\frac{1}{m} \left[\Sigma_{i=1}^{m} \Sigma_{j=1}^{k} 1 \left\{ y^{(i)} = j \right\} \log \frac{e^{\theta_j^T x^{(i)}}}{\Sigma_{\ell=1}^{k} e^{\theta_\ell^T x^{(i)}}} \right], \tag{1}$$

where 1{.} is the indicator function, so that 1{a true statement} = 1, and 1{a false statement} = 0.

3   Experiment

3.1   Dataset Preparation

The lung CT images used in this paper were downloaded from the online resource named LIDC-IDRI [3], in which the malignancy assessments are defined in five levels, i.e., 1, 2, 3, 4, and 5, from benign to malignant. In this study, those nodules labeled "1" and "2" were as benign class, and the rest were as malignant nodules. The final dataset contains 5820 images, training set (60%), validation set (15%) and test set (25%).

3.2   Experiments Design and Analysis

A number of comparison experiments will be demonstrated for validation, and the Receiver Operating Characteristics (ROC) Curve and the Area Under Curve (AUC) are exploited to testify the accuracy of the model. The dimension of full connection layer $n_h = \{100, 500, 1000\}$, the kernel size $n_s = \{3, 5, 7\}$, the number $n_c = \{48, 96, 144\}$, the results were used to examine which network structure was more effective. The models as mentioned above were implemented on the keras[1] deep learning framework. The HOG and LBP features are extracted based on the scikit-image [5] and the proposed models are trained by the GPU (NVIDIA Tesla K80).

At the beginning of either multi-branch or multi-channel pipeline, it needs to calculate the LBP and HOG feature maps as the input. As shown in Table.1, the experimental result indicates that the models respectively performed very well when the HOG parameters with Cell_size = 8, and the LBP with a parameter P = 16 and R = 1. Please note, these results are produced by a general CNN model.

– Multi-Channel CNN model

For the multi-channel feature fusion CNN model in Fig. 2, the gray scale, LBP feature and HOG are trained as the input of CNN, then the accuracy and AUC of the model on the test set are calculated. The experimental results showed that compared with those models by using only the original pulmonary nodule gray scale, by adding the LBP feature map and HOG feature map, the model performs much better. The results show that the accuracy is improved by 0.017 and the AUC is increased by 1.65% compared with by only using the gray scale image as the input (as shown in Figs. 4 and 5).

---

[1] https://github.com/fchollet/keras.

Table 1. Accuracy and AUC for varying HOG and LBP feature parameters

Feature	Parameters' configuration	Accuracy	AUC
HOG	Cell_size = 6	87.84	0.9417
	Cell_size = 8	*89.61*	*0.9510*
	Cell_size = 10	88.93	0.9420
LBP	P = 12, R = 1	86.40	0.9321
	P = 16, R = 1	*89.53*	*0.9512*
	P = 20, R = 1	89.10	0.9410

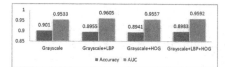

Fig. 4. Accuracy and AUC of varying branching CNN at the same scale

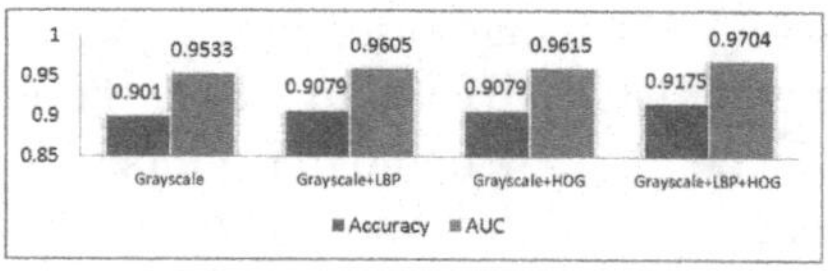

Fig. 5. Accuracy and AUC with varying feature of multi-channel CNN

– Comparison Among Models

In order to visualize the advantages of each algorithm, the outputted features for each model are reduced to three dimensions by t-SNE [8] algorithm, and the MATPLOTLIB library[2] of python is used to plot their spatial distribution patterns. (as shown in Fig. 6). It can be seen from the figures that the CNN models after feature fusion have much gains in the discrimination of benign and malignant lung nodules compared to the conventional CNN model. The CNN model with the multi-channel CNN model has the best differentiation, and the multi-branch CNN Model followed. The ROC curves of the three models are shown in Fig. 7, the dashed line represents the traditional CNN models, the cyan indicates the CNN models of the multi-channel feature fusion, and the blue represent the CNN models of the branching feature fusion. In summary, the feature fusion CNN model has a much better performance.

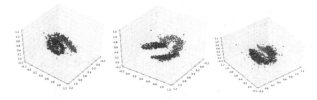

Fig. 6. Feature distribution: left is the plot for the conventional CNN, middle is for multi-branch CNN and right is the plot of multi-channel CNN

---

[2] http://matplotlib.org/.

Table 2. Accuracy and AUC of different models: the blue stands for the results given in the original literature

Feature extraction method	Classifier	Accuracy	AUC
2D Texture [7]	SVM-RBF	87.5	0.942
3D Texture [7]	SVM-RBF	–	*0.9441*
Auto-encoder [9]	Decision Tree	82.68	–
MC-CNN [13]	Softmax	*87.14*	*0.93*
The proposed model	Softmax	*91.75*	*0.9704*

We also compared the differentiation method of lung nodules in literature with our method, and the results are shown in Table 2. The tabular shows that our method outperforms those traditional methods previous presented.

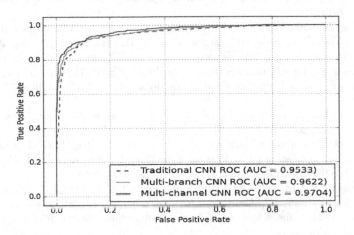

Fig. 7. ROC for conventional CNN model and feature fusion CNN models (Color figure online)

4 Conclusion

In this paper, we proposed a hybrid CNN model for CT images of pulmonary nodules, and improved it through multi-feature fusion to solve the differentiation of benign and malignant for pulmonary nodules. The comparative experiments show that the hybrid fusion CNN model outperforms those methods presented before. After a multi-channel feature fusion,the model can combine the LBP feature and HOG feature to capture the significant feature information of benign and malignant pulmonary nodules more effectively. Although deep learning has strong self-learning ability,the traditional feature integration model can strengthen the important feature information in the initial stage to improve the classification accuracy.

References

1. Anirudh, R., Thiagarajan, J.J., Bremer, P., Kim, H.: Lung nodule detection using 3D convolutional neural networks trained on weakly labeled data. In: Proceedings of SPIE, p. 978532 (2016)
2. Anthimopoulos, M., Christodoulidis, S., Ebner, L., Christe, A., Mougiakakou, S.: Lung pattern classification for interstitial lung diseases using a deep convolutional neural network. IEEE Trans. Med. Imaging 35(5), 1207–1216 (2016)
3. Armato, S.G., Mclennan, G., Bidaut, L., Mcnittgray, M.F., Meyer, C.R., Reeves, A.P., Zhao, B., Aberle, D.R., Henschke, C.I., Hoffman, E.A., et al.: The lung image database consortium (LIDC) and image database resource initiative (IDRI) a completed reference database of lung nodules on CT scans. Med. Phys. 38(2), 915–931 (2011)
4. Dalal, N., Triggs, B.: Histograms of oriented gradients for human detection, vol. 1, pp. 886–893 (2005)
5. Der Walt, S.V., Schonberger, J.L., Nuneziglesias, J., Boulogne, F., Warner, J.D., Yager, N., Gouillart, E., Yu, T.: Scikit-image: image processing in python. PeerJ 2, e453 (2014)
6. Gutierrez, D.: Cancer Facts and Figures. American Family Physician (2015)
7. Han, F., Wang, H., Song, B., Zhang, G., Lu, H., Moore, W., Liang, Z., Zhao, H.: Efficient 3d texture feature extraction from CT images for computer-aided diagnosis of pulmonary nodules. In: Proceedings of SPIE (2014)
8. Hinton, G.E.: Visualizing high-dimensional data using T-SNE. Vigiliae Christianae (2008)
9. Kumar, D., Wong, A., Clausi, D.A.: Lung nodule classification using deep features in CT images, pp. 133–138 (2015)
10. Ludwig, O., Delgado, D., Goncalves, V., Nunes, U.: Trainable classifier-fusion schemes: an application to pedestrian detection. In: International IEEE Conference on Intelligent Transportation Systems, pp. 1–6 (2009)
11. Macmahon, H., Austin, J.H.M., Gamsu, G., Herold, C.J., Jett, J.R., Naidich, D.P., Patz, E.F., Swensen, S.J.: Guidelines for management of small pulmonary nodules detected on CT scans: a statement from the fleischner society. Radiology 237(2), 395–400 (2005)
12. Ojala, T., Pietikainen, M., Harwood, D.: A comparative study of texture measures with classification based on featured distributions. Pattern Recognit. 29(1), 51–59 (1996)
13. Shen, W., Zhou, M., Yang, F., Yu, D., Dong, D., Yang, C., Zang, Y., Tian, J.: Multi-crop convolutional neural networks for lung nodule malignancy suspiciousness classification. Pattern Recognit. 61, 663–673 (2017)
14. Shin, H., Roth, H.R., Gao, M., Lu, L., Xu, Z., Nogues, I., Yao, J., Mollura, D.J., Summers, R.M.: Deep convolutional neural networks for computer-aided detection: CNN architectures, dataset characteristics and transfer learning. IEEE Trans. Med. Imaging 35(5), 1285–1298 (2016)
15. Wang, X., Han, T.X., Yan, S.: An hog-LBP human detector with partial occlusion handling, pp. 32–39 (2009)

A 3D Ultrasound Informed Model of the Human Gastrocnemius Muscle

M. Alipour[1], K. Mithraratne[1], R.D. Herbert[2], and J. Fernandez[1,3(✉)]

[1] Auckland Bioengineering Institute, University of Auckland, Auckland, New Zealand
j.fernandez@auckland.ac.nz
[2] Neuroscience Research Australia, Sydney, Australia
[3] Department of Engineering Science, University of Auckland, Auckland, NZ, New Zealand

Abstract. Muscle fascicle structure characterises muscle function, which in turn plays a key role in computer simulation of muscle shape. In this study we use 3D ultrasound from human gastrocnemius muscle to identify and map the muscle fascicle orientation and deformation during passive motion in four subjects. This muscle fascicle description is integrated into a representative muscle volume element using a free-form deformation technique to create a muscle primitive that deforms according to the embedded muscle fascicles within. For each subject computed passive tensile force was used to optimise the constitutive behaviour so that the known deformation matched this load. Each subject was fit to match deformation at 25%, 50%, 75% and 100% of muscle stretch. The medial gastrocnemius muscle built from these muscle primitives exhibited a contractile shape that is consistent to that observed in human gastrocnemius contraction. This shape was evaluated against the same muscle embedded with muscle fascicles derived from diffusion-weighted magnetic resonance imaging and was in good qualitative agreement. Muscle primitives may be used as building blocks to build large muscle volumes for mechanics simulation, visualisation and medical education.

Keywords: Finite elements · Gastrocnemius · Ultrasound · Muscle mechanics

1 Introduction

Muscle fascicle architecture has been reported as a key factor in how well continuum computer models predict muscle shape and muscle force. For example, the detailed muscle fascicle architecture of the myocardium was reported by Nielsen et al. [1] who showed how contractile function is highly dictated by 3 microstructural directions. Material properties were fitted to the 'pole-zero' constitutive strain energy density function [2] which is also adopted in this study. Skeletal muscle continuum fascicle descriptions play a key role in understanding physiological behaviour as part of multiscale models. Whole continuum muscle behaviour is highly influenced from homogenising substructural models that contain detailed muscle fascicle descriptions [3]. Further, the orientation of muscle fascicles fitted to continuum FE models has been shown to explain the non-uniform strains observed in experiment [4].

© Springer International Publishing AG 2017
M.J. Cardoso et al. (Eds.): BIVPCS/POCUS 2017, LNCS 10549, pp. 27–34, 2017.
DOI: 10.1007/978-3-319-67552-7_4

Including muscle fascicles within a FE framework should not be linked to a specific element type but rather fitted to a mesh topology. One possible approach is to use a NURBS description and integrate this with a FEM (finite element model) for generic elements [5]. In this study we adopt a similar approach whereby a discrete muscle fascicle data set is fitted to a continuum field using a basis function that describes the element interpolation (from linear to cubic). Muscle fascicle vectors are treated as a continuous field that may be applied to any element type. Basic building blocks serve as an efficient way to construct whole muscle volumes. For example a brick element basis with embedded muscle fascicles has been used to construct an entire cat gastrocnemius [6] and was shown to agree with experimental measurement of muscle deformations and force. Moreover, the concept of embedding digitised cadaver muscle fascicle fields into FE model primitives has been presented before [7], which can improve predicted force and contractile shape by up to 20% over simplified parallel muscle fascicle fields.

Ultrasound is a real-time imaging modality used widely to assess size and pennation of muscles such as in the quadriceps of young and old women [8] and *in vivo* pennation angle in human quadriceps [9]. Specific muscle fascicle behaviour has also been evaluated including the relationships between muscle fascicle size and angle [10], changes in pennation with joint angle and torque [11], prediction of tibialis anterior pennation angle changes during dorsiflexion [12]; and the *in vivo* human gastrocnemius architecture during rest and isometric contraction [13].

In this study we extend this concept by deriving a FE primitive from *in vivo* 3D ultrasound data from passive deformation of the human gastrocnemius. The model is developed for four subjects to predict deformation in a representative volume of interest (a muscle element primitive) as part of a FE analysis. For each subject the passive tensile force was measured and combined with the fascicular data to determine subject-specific passive constitutive muscle parameters. The model was fit to 25%, 50%, 75% and 100% muscle deformation for each subject. A medial gastrocnemius muscle is built from these muscle primitives to highlight usability. Contractile mechanics simulations are run to observe predicted surface shape. Ultrasound informed muscle shape is compared with an equivalent geometrical model informed with muscle fascicles derived from Diffusion Tensor Imaging (DTI).

2 Methods

2.1 Experiment

The ultrasound data used in this study are a subset of data that have been reported elsewhere [14]. Four subjects (mean age 24.6 ± 5.2, mean weight 60.6 ± 10.8 kg, mean height 171.6 ± 6.4 cm) had 3D ultrasound collected during a passive seated knee flexion task. The knee was flexed about $79 \pm 6.7°$ (Fig. 1).

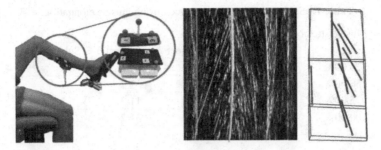

Fig. 1. (Left) Each subject was seated with their leg in a flexed pose and the foot was moved through dorsiflexion. A triad of markers attached to the leg was used to define the leg frame of reference. Markers are also attached to the ultrasound transducer to define the imaging plane. (Middle) 3D Ultrasound image identifying a manually segmented muscle fascicle. (Right) Muscle fascicles embedded inside a three-element 3D host mesh, a FE muscle primitive.

No subjects had any musculoskeletal disorders. Ethical approval was obtained from the South Eastern Sydney Local Health District Human Research Ethics Committee. The left foot was placed on a dynamometer foot plate (Cybex Norm with Humac, CSMi, Stoughton, MA, USA) and the ankle was rotated from fully plantarflexed to fully dorsiflexed. Ankle rotation was slow (5 degrees/second) as slow speed stretches are unlikely to evoke muscle stretch reflexes, so the muscle is more likely to be passive. Surface electromyography (EMG) was used to confirm that the ankle plantarflexor muscles were relaxed. Two ultrasound transducers (Esaote MyLab25 with LA522E 46 mm linear array, 7.5–12 MHz operating at 12 MHz; Esaote, Genoa, Italy) were used synchronously to image the gastrocnemius over the core muscle belly with a field of view of 110 mm. The location and orientation of the ultrasound image in leg space was determined using an optical 3D motion analysis system. For full ultrasound experiment protocols see the work of Herbert et al. [14]. Passive tensile force T_m in the gastrocnemius muscle was computed using the method described by Hoang and colleagues [15]. This involved measuring the passive torque-angle relationship of the ankle at a range of knee angles. Changes in the passive torque-angle relationship of the ankle with knee angle were assumed to be due solely to the two-joint gastrocnemius muscle. The plantarflexor muscles were assumed to be relaxed if there was no discernible increase in EMG amplitude above baseline levels (standard practice in human muscle physiology). The weakest contractions that a person can make voluntarily can easily be identified in this way. T_m is related to muscle length by Eq. 1 with details given in Kwah et al. [16].

$$T_m = \frac{1}{\alpha_G} e^{\alpha_G(\text{lg}-\text{lgs})} \tag{1}$$

where α_G is a constant, found by optimisation, that determines the stiffness of the muscle and is referred to as the "stiffness index" [16]. *lg* is the muscle length and *lgs* the muscle slack length. For all the tensile forces collected, see Tables 1 and 2.

Table 1. Subject passive tensile force during muscle elongation.

Muscle stretch %	Tensile force (N)			
	Subject 1	Subject 2	Subject 3	Subject 4
25.00%	1.5	2.8	0.8	0.3
50.00%	4.1	8.4	3.7	1.7
75.00%	8.5	19.6	11.3	6.3
100.00%	15.5	39.9	31.7	21.1

Table 2. Min/max tensile force, Min/max muscle length, muscle slack length and muscle stiffness index for each subject.

	Subject 1	Subject 2	Subject 3	Subject 4
Tensile force min (N)	2.5	1.9	0.4	0.1
Tensile force max (N)	42.4	17.5	32.1	21.2
Muscle length min (m)	0.38	0.406	0.392	0.394
Muscle length max (m)	0.42	0.431	0.428	0.439
Muscle stiffness index (m^{-1})	82.8	88.6	127.2	119.4
Slack length (m)	0.3	0.3	0.4	0.4

2.2 Finite Element Model

For each subject a set of muscle fascicles were digitised by identifying the 3D coordinates of the muscle fascicles' origins and insertions into the tendon.

Figure 2 shows this process from the 3D ultrasound set identifying segmented muscle fascicles at 0% elongation. This is repeated for nine muscle fascicles with the proximal and distal insertions shown as spheres. Finally, the muscle fascicles are embedded inside a three-element host mesh, which represents the basic muscle primitive in this study. This primitive is morphed so as to minimise the distance between green landmarks and red targets. In order to solve this we employ an iterative closest point algorithm to solve a least squares minimisation. The objective function that is minimised is:

$$F(u_n) = \sum_{d=1}^{N} W_d ||u(\xi_{1d}, \xi_{2d}, \xi_{3d}) - z_d||^2 + F_s(u_n) \tag{2}$$

where z_d are the geometric coordinates of the target points for the muscle fascicle d, w_d is a weighting for each control point, $u(\xi_{1d}, \xi_{2d}, \xi_{3d})$ are the landmark points interpolated at the finite element material coordinates $(\xi_{1d}, \xi_{2d}, \xi_{3d})$ and $F_s(u_n)$ is the Sobolev smoothing penalty function [17] used to conserve muscle primitive volume. A structurally based orthotropic constitutive law previously used for passive cardiac [18] and skeletal muscle [19], the 'pole-zero' relation [2] was adopted and is defined in Eq. 3

$$W = k_{\alpha\beta} \frac{E_{\alpha\beta}^2}{\left| a_{\alpha\beta} \, E_{\alpha\beta} \right|^{b_{\alpha\beta}}} \tag{3}$$

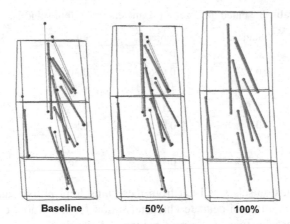

Fig. 2. Free form deformation of subject 1 highlighting the matching of all baseline muscle fascicles to the muscle fascicle locations at 50% and 100% elongation. This produces a deformed host whose shape minimises the difference between baseline and target muscle fascicles.

where the strain energy density function, W, is defined by an asymptote function with $k_{\alpha\beta}$ the scaling function, $b_{\alpha\beta}$ curvature control, $a_{\alpha\beta}$ a strain limiting pole and $E_{\alpha\beta}$ the Green's strain components. The model was treated as transversely isotropic with the muscle fascicle direction $\alpha = \beta = 1$ aligned to the muscle fascicle orientation from ultrasound images. After choosing an initial guess for the 'pole-zero' law we optimised parameters that minimised the difference between the measured muscle tensile force and the computed tensile force. This was performed until the RMS error was less than 0.01 N (or $0.58 \pm 0.19\%$ error across all subjects). For this study we optimised the pole ($a_{\alpha\beta}$) in the muscle fascicle direction, which was the most sensitive parameter and fixed the scaling ($k_{\alpha\beta}$) and curvature ($b_{\alpha\beta}$) parameters. The curvature was set to 1.0 and scaling coefficient set to 0.1 MPa based on previous investigations with cardiac [2] and skeletal tissues [19]. We set a bound on the solution space for $a_{\alpha\beta}$ as 0.01 to 5.0. All models were simulated using the custom software, CMISS, available at www.cmiss.org.

3 Results

Following optimisation of the muscle fascicle end points to match 25% to 100% of muscle stretch the deformed host shape was predicted. The average RMS error between landmark and target muscle fascicles was at most 2 mm in all host mesh deformations. The constitutive law was fit for all four subjects with parameters given in Table 3.

Table 3. Fitted 'pole zero' parameters for all four subjects.

	Subject 1	Subject 2	Subject 3	Subject 4
scaling κ_{11} (MPa)	0.1	0.1	0.1	0.1
pole α_{11}	0.12755	0.656	0.3047	0.494
curvature β_{11}	1	1	1	1
scaling κ_{22}/κ_{33} (MPa)	0.1	0.1	0.1	0.1
pole α_{22}/α_{33}	0.8	0.8	0.8	0.8
curvature β_{22}/β_{33}	1	1	1	1
Avg % error	0.73%	0.71%	0.56%	0.30%

A gastrocnemius muscle was built from these muscle primitives and is shown in
Fig. 3. There was a clear bi-pennate characterisation for the whole continuum with
muscle fascicles merging towards a central tendon. A finite elastic mechanics simulation
using a Hill type contraction model produced a distinct bulge on the medial head of the
gastrocnemius (the larger head) and a distinct crease formed between the heads. To
evaluate this behaviour we compared this with the same muscle fitted with DTI derived
muscle fascicles under the same level of contraction and the resulting muscle profile
was highly consistent with an RMS error difference in shape of 8.8 mm.

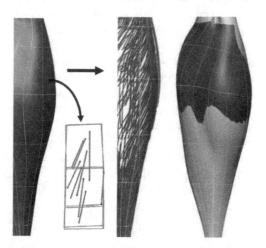

Fig. 3. (Left) Medial gastrocnemius muscle constructed from FE primitive. (Middle) Embedded
muscle fibres. (Right) Fully contracted muscle derived from ultrasound (red) overlaid on same
geometry with diffusion tensor imaging derived fibres (gold). (Color figure online)

4 Discussion

The study developed a muscle primitive using 3D ultrasound in the human gastrocnemius from four subjects as a representation of a bipennate muscle. The extracted 3D
ultrasound muscle fascicle data were embedded inside a representative muscle volume
element that captured approximately 4 cm × 2 cm × 2 cm of the muscle belly and

morphed to match the moving muscle fascicle field imaged from 3D ultrasound using a free-form deformation technique called 'host-mesh' fitting. This produced a series of known muscle shapes (that matched the underlying muscle fascicle data) and we mechanically simulated these known displacements in order to match the measured muscle tensile force by optimising material properties. The 'pole-zero' parameters were optimised to match four positions in the data (25%, 50%, 75% and 100%) of the experimental passive muscle stretch with an average fitting error of less than 1% of the tensile force. It was shown that the whole continuum muscle produced a realistic contractile shape when simulated, which was comparable with a DTI derived model. These muscle primitives are being developed as part of the Physiome repository [19] and the Musculoskeletal Atlas Project (MAP) [20] in order for people to adopt and fit to subject-specific data.

It was observed that the benefit of modelling muscle volume at the chose scale was that all the muscle fascicle and muscle fascicle connection behaviour is captured in the one muscle primitive. Hence, the scale of the representative muscle element is highly suitable as a building block for whole muscles without being concerned about multiscale methods, which is more computationally challenging. Future uses of this data include characterising healthy versus pathologic muscle and creating a table of material parameters for patients with different age and health conditions to be used for mechanics and graphical representation.

References

1. Nielsen, P., et al.: Mathematical model of geometry and fibrous structure of the heart. Am. J. Physiol. Heart Circ. Physiol. **260**(4), H1365–H1378 (1991)
2. Hunter, P.J.: Myocardial constitutive laws for continuum mechanics models of the heart. In: Sideman, S., Beyar, R. (eds.) Molecular and Subcellular Cardiology. Advances in Experimental Medicine and Biology, vol. 382, pp. 303–318. Springer, Boston (1995)
3. Röhrle, O., et al.: A physiologically based, multi-scale model of skeletal muscle structure and function. Frontiers Physiol. **3**, 358 (2012)
4. Blemker, S.S., et al.: A 3D model of muscle reveals the causes of nonuniform strains in the biceps brachii. J. Biomech. **38**(4), 657–665 (2005)
5. Lu, Y., et al.: Modelling skeletal muscle fibre orientation arrangement. Comput. Methods Biomechan. Biomed. Eng. **14**(12), 1079–1088 (2011)
6. Lemos, R., et al.: A framework for structured modeling of skeletal muscle. Comput. Methods Biomech. Biomed. Eng. **7**(6), 305–317 (2004)
7. Sánchez, C.A., et al.: Embedding digitized fibre fields in finite element models of muscles. Comput. Methods Biomech. Biomed. Eng. Imaging Vis. **2**(4), 223–236 (2014)
8. Young, A., et al.: Size and strength of the quadriceps muscles of old and young women*. Eur. J. Clin. Invest. **14**(4), 282–287 (1984)
9. Rutherford, O., et al.: Measurement of fibre pennation using ultrasound in the human quadriceps in vivo. Eur. J. Appl. Physiol. **65**(5), 433–437 (1992)
10. Henriksson-Larsen, K., et al.: Do muscle fibre size and fibre angulation correlate in pennated human muscles? Eur. J. Appl. Physiol. **64**(1), 68–72 (1992)
11. Herbert, R., et al.: Changes in pennation with joint angle and muscle torque: in vivo measurements in human brachialis muscle. J. Physiol. **484**(Pt 2), 523–532 (1995)

12. Maganaris, C.N., et al.: Predictability of in vivo changes in pennation angle of human tibialis anterior muscle from rest to maximum isometric dorsiflexion. Eur. J. Appl. Physiol. **79**(3), 294–297 (1999)
13. Narici, M., et al.: In vivo human gastrocnemius architecture with changing joint angle at rest and during graded isometric contraction. J. Physiol. **496**(Pt. 1), 287–297 (1996)
14. Herbert, R., et al.: Changes in the length and three-dimensional orientation of muscle fascicles and aponeuroses with passive length changes in human gastrocnemius muscles. J. Physiol. **593**(2), 441–455 (2015)
15. Hoang, P.D., et al.: A new method for measuring passive length-tension properties of human gastrocnemius muscle in vivo. J. Biomech. **38**(6), 1333–1341 (2005)
16. Kwah, L.K., et al.: Passive mechanical properties of gastrocnemius muscles of people with ankle contracture after stroke. Arch. Phys. Med. Rehabil. **93**(7), 1185–1190 (2012)
17. Fernandez, J.W., et al.: Anatomically based geometric modelling of the musculo-skeletal system and other organs. Biomech. Model. Mechanobiol. **2**(3), 139–155 (2004)
18. Hunter, P., et al.: Modelling the mechanical properties of cardiac muscle. Prog. Biophys. Mol. Biol. **69**(2), 289–331 (1998)
19. Fernandez, J., et al.: Modelling the passive and nerve activated response of the rectus femoris muscle to a flexion loading: a finite element framework. Med. Eng. Phys. **27**(10), 862–870 (2005)
20. Zhang, J., et al.: The MAP client: user-friendly musculoskeletal modelling workflows. In: Bello, F., Cotin, S. (eds.) ISBMS 2014. LNCS, vol. 8789, pp. 182–192. Springer, Cham (2014). doi:10.1007/978-3-319-12057-7_21

Atlas-Based 3D Intensity Volume Reconstruction of Musculoskeletal Structures in the Lower Extremity from 2D Calibrated X-Ray Images

Weimin Yu[✉] and Guoyan Zheng

Institute for Surgical Technology and Biomechanics,
University of Bern, Bern, Switzerland
weimin.yu@istb.unibe.ch

Abstract. In this paper, the reconstruction of 3D intensity volumes of femur, tibia and three muscles around the thigh region from a pair of calibrated X-ray images is addressed. We present an atlas-based 2D-3D intensity volume reconstruction approach by combining a 2D-2D non-rigid registration based 3D landmark reconstruction procedure with an adaptive regularization step. More specifically, an atlas derived from the CT acquisition of a healthy lower extremity, together with the input calibrated X-ray images are used to reconstruct those musculoskeletal structures. To avoid the potential penetration of the reconstructed femoral and tibial volumes that might be caused by reconstruction error, we come up with an articulated 2D-3D reconstruction strategy, which can effectively preserve knee joint structure. Another contribution from our work is the application of the proposed 2D-3D reconstruction pipeline to derive the patient-specific volumes of three thigh muscles around the thigh region.

Keywords: Atlas · 2D-3D reconstruction · Articulated · Lower extremity · Musculoskeletal

1 Introduction

In order to reduce radiation exposure to patients, 2D-3D reconstruction, which can reconstruct 3D patient-specific models from 2D X-ray images, is proposed as an alternative to CT scan for certain applications. Depending on the output, those 2D-3D reconstruction methods can be generally classified into two categories [1]: 3D surface model reconstruction [2,3] and 3D intensity volume reconstruction [4–7]. The methods in the former category compute 3D patient-specific surface models from one or multiple 2D X-ray images. No intensity information or information about cortical bone is available. The methods in the second category generate 3D patient-specific volumes from a limited number of X-ray images. Most of the previous work tried to solve the ill-posed problem of 2D-3D volume reconstruction by introducing different statistical prior models, while Yu et al. [7] firstly explored the potential of atlas-based 2D-3D intensity volume

© Springer International Publishing AG 2017
M.J. Cardoso et al. (Eds.): BIVPCS/POCUS 2017, LNCS 10549, pp. 35–43, 2017.
DOI: 10.1007/978-3-319-67552-7_5

reconstruction. To our knowledge, none of the above mentioned methods have been applied to reconstruct the intensity volumes of a complete lower extremity.

In this paper we present an atlas-based 2D-3D intensity volume reconstruction approach which is an extension of the previous work [7] and we apply it to reconstruct 3D intensity volumes of femur, tibia and three muscles around the thigh region from a pair of 2D X-ray images.

The remainder of the paper is arranged as follows: the techniques of the proposed atlas-based 2D-3D reconstruction method will be described in Sect. 2. Section 3 will present the results of our validation experiments on several datasets, followed by the discussions and conclusions in Sect. 4.

2   Materials and Methods

2.1   Atlas Preparation

The atlas consists of the template volumes of femur and tibia as well as the template volumes of rectus femoris muscle, vastus lateralis & intermedius muscle, and vastus medialis muscle (if reconstructing these thigh muscles) which are segmented from the CT data of a healthy lower extremity. In addition, the atlas includes two sets of sparse 3D landmarks ($\{L_{femur,n}\}_{n=1}^{N_1}$ and $\{L_{tibia,n}\}_{n=1}^{N_2}$) extracted from the outer surfaces and the intramedullary canal surfaces of the template volumes.

2.2   The 2D-3D Reconstruction Pipeline

The 2D-3D reconstruction process is aiming to fit the atlas to a pair of X-ray images, one acquired from the Anterior-Posterior (AP) direction and the other from a oblique view (not necessary the Lateral-Medial (LM) direction). Both images are calibrated and co-registered to a common coordinate system called **c**. A template volume $I(x)$ is aligned to the reference space **c** via a forward mapping: $I(x_c(T_g, T_d)) = I(T_g \circ T_d \circ x_f)$, where x_f is a point in the template space. Here, a global scaled-rigid transformation T_g as well as a local deformation T_d are to be determined via a 2D-3D scaled-rigid registration stage and a 2D-3D intensity volume reconstruction stage. Both stages are based on the procedure of 2D-2D non-rigid registration based 3D landmark reconstruction.

The 2D-2D non-rigid registration based 3D landmark reconstruction follows the previous work [7] which is organized in a hierarchical style: (1) Digitally reconstructed radiography (DRR) generation and 3D landmark projection; (2) non-rigid 2D-2D intensity-based registration; and (3) triangulation-based landmark reconstruction. Inspired by the work [2], 3D sparse landmarks instead of the B-Spline control points used in the previous work are adapted.

Given the initial transformation of the template volumes to the common coordinate system **c** via landmark-based alignment, we can generate virtual 2D radiographic images and also project those 3D sparse landmarks. The non-rigid 2D deformation fields obtained from the registration module based on the registration library "elastix" [8] enable us to look for the dimensional correspondences represented by the paired 2D projected landmarks, and then new 3D sparse landmarks are reconstructed via the triangulation which is in several milliseconds for each landmark reconstruction.

2D-3D Scaled-Rigid Alignment is conducted via the paired-point matching between the reconstructed 3D landmarks and the original 3D landmarks in the atlas (see Fig. 1, left), and we iteratively compute $\left\{T_g^t\right\}_{t=1,2,3,\ldots}$ in order to handle those complicated pose differences. The 2D-3D similarity alignment is applied to femur and tibia individually, and finally we can obtain two scaled-rigid transformations T_g^{femur} and T_g^{tibia}. Figure 1, right shows an example of the 2D-3D scaled-rigid alignment which can handle large pose difference.

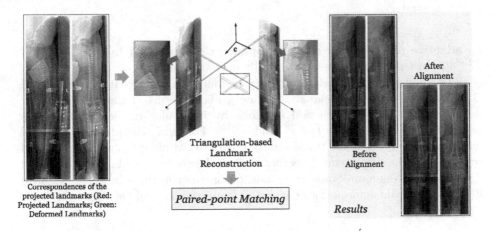

Correspondences of the
projected landmarks (Red:
Projected Landmarks; Green:
Deformed Landmarks)

Triangulation-based
Landmark
Reconstruction

Paired-point Matching

After
Alignment

Before
Alignment

Results

Fig. 1. An illustration of 2D-3D scaled-rigid alignment.

2D-3D Intensity Volume Reconstruction starts with the reconstructed 3D sparse landmarks ($\{L'_{femur,n}\}_{n=1}^{N_1}$ or $\{L'_{tibia,n}\}_{n=1}^{N_2}$) and the original 3D landmarks in the atlas ($\{L_{femur,n}\}_{n=1}^{N_1}$ or $\{L_{tibia,n}\}_{n=1}^{N_2}$). Firstly, we transform these reconstructed landmarks back to the space of the atlas with $T_g^{-1,femur}$ and $T_g^{-1,tibia}$, and then two local deformations T_l^{femur} and T_l^{tibia} can be computed using 3D thin-plate-spline (TPS) transformation as follows:

$$\begin{cases} T_l^{femur} \leftarrow T_{TPS}\left(\{L_{femur,n}\}_{n=1}^{N_1}, \{T_g^{-1,femur} \circ L'_{femur,n}\}_{n=1}^{N_1}\right) \\ T_l^{tibia} \leftarrow T_{TPS}\left(\{L_{tibia,n}\}_{n=1}^{N_2}, \{T_g^{-1,tibia} \circ L'_{tibia,n}\}_{n=1}^{N_2}\right) \end{cases} \quad (1)$$

Notice that the obtained transformations T_l^{femur} and T_l^{tibia} are usually ill-posed since there is no restriction on the behaviors of 3D deformation fields, which may lead to poor reconstruction results (see Fig. 2). Therefore, we apply

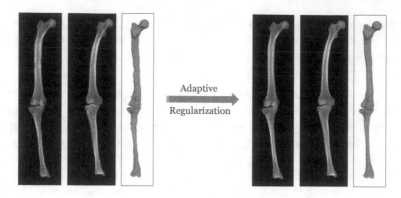

Fig. 2. A comparison of the reconstruction of femur and tibia w/o the adaptive regularization strategy.

an adaptive regularization on the B-Spline grid(s) sampled from T_l^{femur} and T_l^{tibia} in order to derive the anatomically correct results.

The adaptive regularization strategy begins with the layout of a combined B-Spline grid or two individual B-Spline grids in terms of the articulated or individual 2D-3D reconstruction methods by interpolating the displacements at the control points from T_l^{femur} and T_l^{tibia}. Following the previous work [9] which proposed a B-spline transformation regularization approach for non-rigid registration, the displacement vectors d_{ijk} at the control points are regularized based on the Neumann boundary condition on the control points [10]. Figure 3 illustrates the 3D deformations computed from each step of the regularization.

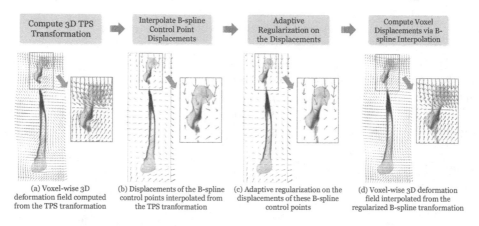

Fig. 3. A comparison of the deformation fields derived from a TPS transformation and from the regularized B-Spline transformation.

In order to prevent the reconstructed femur and tibia from penetrating each other, we investigated two strategies to reconstruct the associated structures:

I. <u>Individual 2D-3D Reconstruction</u>: The reconstruction of femur and tibia is completely individual, and each time just one anatomy will be reconstructed. As indicated, there is no consideration over the articulation of knee joint.

II. <u>Articulated 2D-3D Reconstruction</u>: A combined B-spline grid is placed over the space of the template volumes, and the displacement d_{ijk} at a control point $\mathbf{C}_{ijk}$ is computed either by T_l^{femur} or by T_l^{tibia}, depending on the relative position between a pre-defined axis-aligned plane ζ (see Fig. 4, left) and $\mathbf{C}_{ijk}$:

$$\begin{cases} if\ \mathbf{C}_{ijk}\ is\ above\ \zeta,\ d_{ijk} \leftarrow T_l^{femur}\ (\mathbf{C}_{ijk}) \\ if\ \mathbf{C}_{ijk}\ is\ below\ \zeta,\ d_{ijk} \leftarrow T_l^{tibia}\ (\mathbf{C}_{ijk}) \end{cases} \qquad (2)$$

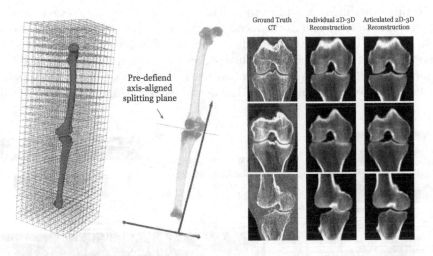

Fig. 4. The schematic view of the articulated 2D-3D reconstruction method (Left) and the qualitative comparison with the individual 2D-3D reconstruction method (Right).

We found that there is basically the same for the reconstruction accuracy from both strategies, while the qualitative comparison of reconstructing knee joint structure demonstrates the superiority of the articulated 2D-3D reconstruction method over the individual one (see Fig. 4, right).

The Reconstruction of Three Muscles Around the Thigh Region: The obtained 3D deformation fields from the reconstruction pipeline provide the potential of reconstructing the muscles in the thigh region. Currently, we just focus on the reconstruction of (1) rectus femoris muscle; (2) vastus lateralis & intermedius muscle; and (3) vastus medialis muscle.

3   Experiments and Results

Approved by a local institution review board (IRB), we conducted three experiments to validate the proposed reconstruction pipeline in regard to different motivations.

3.1   Experiment on CT Dataset of 11 Cadaveric Legs

Each CT data has a voxel spacing of $0.78\,\text{mm} \times 0.78\,\text{mm} \times 1\,\text{mm}$, and we chosen a healthy CT data from them to create the atlas for all experiments. For the atlas, we segmented the binary labels of the femoral and tibial structures as well as their cortical bone regions, and 641 landmarks for femur and 872 landmarks for tibia were extracted from these binary labels.

In this experiment, we'd like to evaluate the overall reconstruction accuracy of femur and tibia as well as the reconstruction accuracy of their intramedullary canal regions. Therefore, for the left 10 sets of CT volumes, we segmented the binary labels of the femoral and tibial structures as well as their cortical bone regions for each CT data as the ground truth, and also we generated a pair of virtual 2D radiographic images (DRRs) as the reference images (see Fig. 5, top).

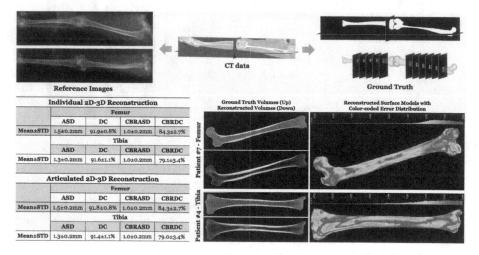

Fig. 5. The reference images & the ground truth from each CT data (Top); and the quantitative (Bottom, Left) and qualitative (Bottom, Right) results of the experiment conducted on 10 cadaveric legs

We assessed both the individual and the articulated 2D-3D reconstruction strategies, and the results are shown in Fig. 5, left. Here, the average surface distance (ASD) and the dice coefficient (DC) for the overall reconstruction and the reconstruction of cortical bone region (i.e. cortical bone region ASD (CBRASD) and cortical bone region DC (CBRDC)) were measured. From the results, there is no statistically significant difference in accuracy but it is distinct in the preservation of knee joint structure from the two strategies (see Fig. 4). Figure 5, right shows a qualitative comparison of the reconstructed volumes with the associated ground truth volumes for both femur and tibia.

3.2   Experiment on X-Ray Images from Patients

10 pairs of X-ray images were collected for this experiment, which is more challenging due to the image quality. Since only the CT data around three local regions (hip, knee and ankle joint) were available, the reconstruction accuracy was evaluated by comparing the surface models extracted from the ground truth CT data with those extracted from the reconstructed volumes after rigidly align them together.

The average surface distance (ASD) for the local regions including proximal femur (PF-ASD), distal femur (DF-ASD), proximal tibia (PT-ASD) and distal tibia (DT-ASD) were measured. The quantitative results are shown in Fig. 6, left where an overall reconstruction accuracy of 1.4 mm was found, and Fig. 6, right shows a reconstruction case.

	#01	#02	#03	#04	#05	#06	#07	#08	#09	#10	Mean±STD
PF-ASD [mm]	1.2	1.2	0.8	0.9	1.3	1.2	1.5	2.2	1.4	0.9	1.3±0.4
DF-ASD [mm]	1.5	1.4	1.5	1.3	1.6	1.9	1.8	1.5	1.4	1.2	1.5±0.2
PT-ASD [mm]	1.1	1.1	1.4	1.2	1.4	1.4	2.2	1.6	1.8	1.4	1.5±0.3
DT-ASD [mm]	1	1.3	1.5	1.5	1.2	1.4	1.5	0.9	1.2	1.5	1.3±0.2

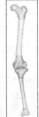

Fig. 6. The average surface distances measured between the reconstructed surface models and the ground truth surface models.

3.3   Experiment on Reconstructing Three Thigh Muscles

We also evaluated the accuracy of reconstructing three thigh muscles on a set of 12 one-side CT data with the associated ground-truth segmentations around the thigh region [11]. One CT volume was randomly chosen to create the atlas, and we conducted the experiment on the left 11 cases. We measured the dice coefficient (DC) to evaluate the reconstruction accuracy of the three thigh muscles, and the results are shown in Fig. 7, ranging from 78% to 85%.

Case	Musculoskeletal Structure Reconstruction – DICE [%]			
	Femur	Rectus Femoris Muscle	Vastus Lateralis & Intermedius Muscle	Vastus Medialis Muscle
#01	93.4	84.6	86.3	74.5
#02	94	85.5	85.8	78.2
#03	90.7	76.2	86.3	80.3
#04	92.8	81.9	82.2	79
#05	90.8	83.4	77.7	74.2
#06	90	71.3	85.5	81.9
#07	89.7	81.3	86	75.3
#08	91.8	77.3	86.1	79.2
#09	92	74	80.1	73.2
#10	90.8	84.6	88.6	79.9
#11	92.4	84.5	88.3	79.8
Overall	91.7±2.4	80.4±4.9	84.8±3.4	77.8±2.9

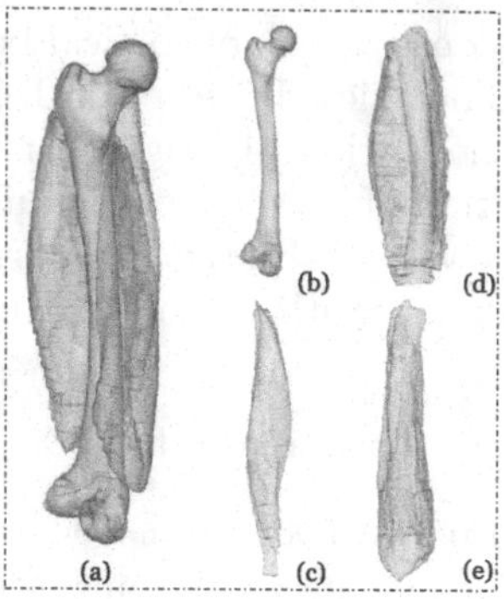

Fig. 7. (a) The femur & thigh muscle reconstruction accuracy: red (ground truth surface) and green (reconstructed surface); (b) femur; (c) rectus femoris muscle; (d) vastus lateralis & intermedius muscle; (e) vastus medialis muscle. (Color figure online)

4   Discussion and Conclusion

We presented an atlas-based 2D-3D intensity volume reconstruction approach, which to our knowledge, is probably the first attempt to derive patient-specific musculoskeletal structures in the lower extremity. Our method has the advantage of combining the robustness of 2D-3D landmark reconstruction with the smoothness properties inherent to B-spline based 3D regularization. In order to preserve knee joint structure, we proposed an articulated 2D-3D reconstruction strategy which can derive the anatomically correct reconstruction results, and we also investigated the reconstruction of three thigh muscles via the proposed reconstruction pipeline, which holds the potential to be used in the clinical routine in future. The comprehensive results from a set of experiments demonstrated the efficacy of this 2D-3D reconstruction method.

References

1. Markelj, P., et al.: A review of 3D/2D registration methods for image-guided interventions. Med. Image Anal. **16**, 642–661 (2012)
2. Zheng, G., et al.: A 2D/3D correspondence building method for reconstruction of a patient-specific 3D bone surface model using point distribution models and calibrated X-ray images. Med. Image Anal. **13**, 883–899 (2009)
3. Baka, N., et al.: 2D–3D reconstruction of the distal femur from stereo X-ray imaging using statistical shape models. Med. Image Anal. **15**, 840–850 (2011)
4. Yao, J., Taylor, R.H.: Assessing accuracy factors in deformable 2D/3D medical image registration using a statistical pelvis model. In: ICCV 2003, pp. 1329–1334 (2003)
5. Ahmad, O., et al.: Volumetric DXA (VXA) - a new method to extract 3D information from multiple in vivo DXA images. J. Bone Miner. Res. **25**, 2468–2475 (2010)

6. Zheng, G.: Personalized X-Ray reconstruction of the proximal femur via intensity-based non-rigid 2D-3D registration. In: Fichtinger, G., Martel, A., Peters, T. (eds.) MICCAI 2011. LNCS, vol. 6892, pp. 598–606. Springer, Heidelberg (2011). doi:10.1007/978-3-642-23629-7_73

7. Yu, W., Chu, C., Tannast, M., Zheng, G.: Fully automatic reconstruction of personalized 3D volumes of the proximal femur from 2D X-ray images. Int. J. Comput. Assist. Radiol. Surg. **11**(9), 1673–1685 (2016)

8. Klein, S., et al.: Elastix: a toolbox for intensity-based medical image registration. IEEE Trans. Med. Imag. **29**(1), 196–205 (2010)

9. Myronenko, A., Song, X.: Adaptive regularization of ill-posed problems: application to non-rigid image registration (2009). arXiv:0906.3323

10. Strang, G.: The discrete cosine transform. SIAM Rev. **41**(1), 135–147 (1999)

11. Chu, C., et al.: Statistical shape modeling of compound musculoskeletal structures around the thigh region. In: ISBI 2016, pp. 885–888 (2016)

Automatic Liver Lesion Segmentation in CT Combining Fully Convolutional Networks and Non-negative Matrix Factorization

Shenhai Zheng[1], Bin Fang[1(✉)], Laquan Li[2], Mingqi Gao[1],
Yi Wang[1], and Kaiyi Peng[1]

[1] College of Computer Science,
Chongqing University, Chongqing 400044, China
fb@cqu.edu.cn
[2] School of Automation, Huazhong University of Science and Technology,
Wuhan 430074, China

Abstract. Automatic liver tumor segmentation is an important step towards digital medical research, clinical diagnosis and therapy planning. However, the existence of noise, low contrast and heterogeneity make the automatic liver tumor segmentation remaining an open challenge. In this work, we focus on a novel automatic method to segment liver tumor in abdomen images from CT scans by using fully convolutional networks (FCN) and non-negative matrix factorization (NMF). We train the FCN for semantic liver and tumor segmentation. The segmented liver and tumor regions of FCN are used as ROI and initialization for the NMF based tumor refinement, respectively. We refine the surfaces of tumors using a 3D deformable model which derived from NMF and driven by local cumulative spectral histograms (LCSH). The refinement is designed to obtain a smoother, more accurate and natural liver tumor surface. Experiments demonstrated that the proposed segmentation method achieves satisfactory results. Likewise, it has been notably observed that the computing time of the segmentation method is no more than one minute for each CT volume.

Keywords: Liver lesion · FCN · Non-negative matrix factorization · Local cumulative spectral histograms · Segmentation

1 Introduction

The liver is a common site of primary or secondary tumor disease development [9]. Segmentation and volume measurement of liver tumors are important tasks for digital medical research, clinical diagnosis and surgical planning. Usually, manual and semi-manual annotation may obtain accurate segmentation results but it is operator-dependent and time-consuming.

With the development of medical imaging, there is an increasing interest in automatic tumor segmentation methods. Due to their variations in the location,

© Springer International Publishing AG 2017
M.J. Cardoso et al. (Eds.): BIVPCS/POCUS 2017, LNCS 10549, pp. 44–51, 2017.
DOI: 10.1007/978-3-319-67552-7_6

appearance and shape, automatic segmentation of liver tumors is very challenging. Until now, many methods have been developed for liver tumors. These methods include the thresholding, graph cuts, watershed, region growing, classification, statistical analysis and so on [12]. Usually, these methods are based on the pixel or voxel intensity which cause boundary leakage, under-segmentation or over-segmentation easily.

To palliate these drawbacks, deformable models [1] have been proven useful in image segmentation due to the sub-pixel accuracy and closed object boundary. Tumor segmentation using active contours [3] and level set [11,17] have been proposed. Some techniques using fuzzy clustering [10] and machine learning [8] methods are also developed. However, these methods are not applied in clinics if there is no user interaction.

To further make the segmentation result plausible, more efficient and robust methods should be involved. Recently, deep convolution neural networks (CNN) are rapidly proven to be the state-of-the-art foundation [14], and achieve enhanced performance in object recognition and segmentation. FCN, based on CNN, has shown impressive results in semantic natural image segmentation [13].

In this work, we focus on the automatic liver tumor segmentation combining FCN and NMF. This combination produces a coarse to fine segmentation pipeline. Firstly, we train the FCN for semantic liver and tumor segmentation. The training data is 116 CT volumes (51247 slices) of LiTS. Secondly, the trained FCN is used to segment liver and tumor regions coarsely. The test data are 3 CT volumes with different tumor size, ambiguous boundary and heterogeneous densities (selected from LiTS and 3D-IRCADb). Thirdly, the segmented tumor is refined by a 3D deformable model within the segmented liver region. The deformable model is derived from NMF and is driven by LCSH. Our contributions are the following: (1) we train and apply FCN on liver and tumor segmentation simultaneously on CT volumes slice by slice (Sect. 2.2), refine the coarse segmentation using 3D deformable model based on (2) LCSP on 3D CT volumes (Sect. 2.3) and (3) NMF (Sect. 2.3).

2   Method

2.1   Overview

Firstly, we present the overview of the proposed segmentation method. The pipeline is shown in Fig. 1 which consist of two parts:

(1) The training part: We train the FCN on the 51247 image slices of LiTS which labeled as background, liver and tumor, respectively.
(2) The segmentation part: Firstly, we use the trained FCN to predict semantic segmentation of input CT volumes slice by slice. The segmented slice are stacked as volumes, and the largest and connected prediction region is selected as ROI. Then, we compute the LCSH on the ROI. Lastly, the surfaces of tumors are refined using the 3D deformable model. The mean LCSH, referred to as representative features, of liver and tumor region within ROI contribute to the initialization of refinement.

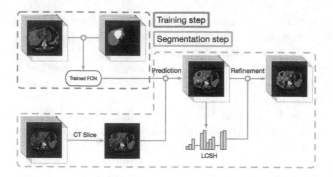

Fig. 1. Pipeline of the proposed liver tumor segmentation method

2.2 FCN

FCNs are a rich class of models that address many pixel-wise tasks. They replace the fully connected layer of classic CNN with convolutional layer and the transposed convolution layer restore the feature map as the size of original image. FCN can solve the semantic segmentation using pixel classification. The motivation behind the semantic liver and liver tumor segmentation using FCN is that many works have demonstrated the generality for a variety of image-to-image tasks. In the proposed method, we trained the FCN based on the configurations network of 19 weight layers of VGGNet [15]. In contrast to the cascaded fully convolutional neural networks [4], the proposed method doesnt have any data augment and pre-processing. And we segment the liver and tumor at once rather than two step segmentation.

During training, we used a PC equipped with a single Core i7-6800K CPU (8 cores, 3.4 GHz) and one NVIDIA GTX 1080 GPU. The framework is tensorflow with a learning rate of 0.0001, a momentum of 0.9 and a batch size of 20.

2.3 Deformable Model

We develop a combined method that uses the FCN to isolate tumor and deformable model to refine the tumor surface from the surrounded parenchyma.

Local Cumulative Spectral Histograms (LCSH): To identify ambiguity boundary between tumor and surrounded liver parenchyma, we present a novel intensity statistical feature using the LCSH. Suppose the gray-scale of CT volume $I : \boldsymbol{x} \in \Omega \rightarrow R$ is $[0, L]$ and Ω_{roi} is ROI ($\Omega_{roi} \subset \Omega$). For a local neighborhood $N(\boldsymbol{x})$ of $\boldsymbol{x}$ in the Ω_{roi}, the LCSH is define by:

$$F_{\boldsymbol{x}}(y_i) = \frac{\#\{\boldsymbol{z} \in N(\boldsymbol{x}) \cap \Omega_{roi} : I(\boldsymbol{z}) \leq y_i\}}{\#\{N(\boldsymbol{x}) \cap \Omega_{roi}\}} \tag{1}$$

$y_i \in [0, L]$ is the largest gray intensity of the ith bin ($i \in \{1, 2, \cdots, N\}$, N is the bin number). And $\#$ denotes the number of elements contained in the set.

Compared to the pixel intensity, LCSH has more power to characterize object, and better ability to suppress noise. Here the image intensity and the response of one LoG filter are used to compute LCSH.

The Segmentation Energy: In most image segmentation methods based on multiple feature maps, the segmentation label is decided through the distance measurement between feature vector and representative feature of each region. But pixels near boundaries are misclassified usually. To address this problem, Yuan et al. [16] proposed a different classification approach using NMF. The segmentation model consider the feature vector of every pixel is a linear combination of the representation features. The segmentation model is given as:

$$Y = RW + \varepsilon \tag{2}$$

where Y is an $N \times M$ feature matrix, R is an $N \times n$ representative feature matrix, W is a $n \times M$ weight matrix and ε is the additive noise. M and n represent the total number of image pixels and segmentation regions. For the given representative features, the weights can be compute as:

$$W = (R^T R)^{-1} R^T Y \tag{3}$$

Then Gao et al. [5] extended the model to the level set framework for texture segmentation. The data fitting energy is expressed as:

$$E(\phi, w_1, w_2) = - \int_\Omega w_1 H(\phi) + w_2 (1 - H(\phi)) d\boldsymbol{x} \tag{4}$$

where w_1 and w_2 are the weight matrix of object and background, respectively. ϕ is level set function and H is the Heaviside function.

In this paper, we propose the 3D segmentation model based on NMF and the LCSH:

$$E(\phi, w_1, w_2) = \int_{\Omega_{roi}} (1 - w_1) H(\phi) + (1 - w_2)(1 - H(\phi)) d\boldsymbol{x} + v \int_{\Omega_{roi}} |\nabla H(\phi)| \, d\boldsymbol{x} \tag{5}$$

v is the weight parameters. The first term is data fidelity energy and the second term is the regularization term. The vectored weight matrix, also denoted by w_1 and w_2, are computed as $(w_1, w_2)^T = (R^T R)^{-1} R^T Y$. In application, the initial representative features R is the mean LCSH of the predicted liver and liver tumor regions by FCN within the ROI.

2.4   Algorithm Implementation

The energy (5) may be minimized by using the gradient descend method. Because of the non-convex, this model prone to different minimum. For the fixed w_1 and w_2, we redefine the energy functional (5) via standard convex minimization schemes [2]. The convex energy $F_G(u)$ is given as:

$$\arg\min_{0 \leq u \leq 1} F_G(u) = \arg\min_{0 \leq u \leq 1} v \int_{\Omega_{roi}} |\nabla u(\boldsymbol{x})| \, d\boldsymbol{x} + \int_{\Omega_{roi}} (w_2 - w_1) u(\boldsymbol{x}) d\boldsymbol{x} \tag{6}$$

We should note that object region is given as $\Omega^*(\mu) = \{x \in \Omega_{roi} | u^* > \mu\}$ where u^* is the global minimizer of the convex energy $F_G(u)$ and $\mu \in (0, 1)$ is a simple thresholding (we set $\mu = 0.5$ in this paper).

Next, we will apply the Split Bregman method [7] to minimize the convex model (6) of u. Introduce the auxiliary variable d such that $d = \nabla u$, the elegant two-phase Split Bregman iteration is given as following:

$$(u^{k+1}, d^{k+1}) = \underset{0 \le u \le 1, d}{\arg \min} v \int_{\Omega_{roi}} |d| \, dx + \int_{\Omega} (w_2 - w_1) u dx + \frac{\gamma}{2} \int_{\Omega} \left\| d - \nabla u - b^k \right\|^2 dx$$
(7)

$$b^{k+1} = b^k + \nabla u^{k+1} - d^{k+1}$$
(8)

The Euler-Lagrange equation of the optimization problem (7) with respect to u is:

$$\Delta u^{k+1} = \frac{w_2 - w_1}{\gamma} + \nabla(d^k - b^k)$$
(9)

Gauss-Seidel formula is used to solve this equation.

Likewise, the optimization problem (7) with respect to d is:

$$d^{k+1} = shrink(\nabla u^{k+1}, \frac{v}{\gamma})$$
(10)

where $shrink(\alpha, \beta)$ is the shrinkage operator defined as:

$$shrink(\alpha, \beta) = \begin{cases} \frac{\alpha}{|\alpha|} \max(|\alpha| - \beta, 0), & \alpha \ne 0 \\ 0, & \alpha \ne 0 \end{cases}$$
(11)

After one iteration, w_1 and w_2 are updated using the representative features R computed by the mean LCSH in $\{x \in \Omega_{roi} | u^{k+1} > \mu\}$ and $\{x \in \Omega_{roi} | u^{k+1} < \mu\}$.

3   Experiments and Result

3.1   Dataset

The tested data come from two public databases 3D-IRCADb and LiTS. The 3D-IRCADb database is composed of 20 CT scans with hepatic tumors in 75% of cases. The LiTS includes 131 training CT scans and 70 test CT scans. The training data were labeled as liver region, tumor or background. CT scans of these two public databases differ substantially among the level of contrast, number and size of tumor tumors. Slice numbers of all the CT volumes vary from 64 to 987. The inner/inter-slice pixel spacing is 0.56~1/0.7~5 mm. Without loss of generality, in this paper, we select 3 CT volumes (no. 3 and 4 of LiTS, no.19 of 3D-IRCADb) with different tumor size, ambiguous boundary and heterogeneous densities to demonstrate the efficiency of the proposed method.

3.2 Evaluation Criteria

In order to evaluate the proposed segmentation method, five measures [9], namely Volumetric Overlap Error (VOE, %), Relative Volume Difference (RVD, %), Average Symmetric Surface Distance (ASD, mm), Root Mean Square Symmetric Surface Distance (RMSD, mm), Maximum Symmetric Surface Distance (MSD, mm), are used for segmentation evaluation. For these measures, the smaller the (absolute) value is, the better the segmentation result is. Particularly, zero for all the five measures denotes a perfect segmentation. Other three correct evaluation metrics [6] (Sensitivity, Specificity and Accuracy) are used. For the three metrics, the bigger the value ([0, 1]) is, the better the segmentation result is.

3.3 Results and Analysis

In this subsection, firstly, we visually compared the proposed method with fuzzy clustering method (FLICM) [10] and level set approach (LSACM) [17] on 2D case with the predicted liver mask of FCN. The results reveal that our method outperforms the other compared methods.

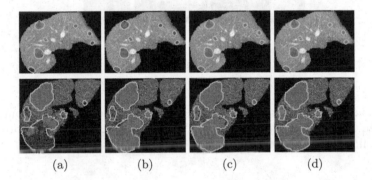

Fig. 2. Comparison results on 2D case. (a) FCN, (b) FLICM, (c) LSACM, and (d) The proposed. The segmentation results are shown with green mask and the ground truths are surround by yellow contour. (Color figure online)

Then, we evaluate the proposed method on the selected three data. In Fig. 3, typical 3D distance map between the segmented tumors and ground truth are visually represented. Quantitative evaluation results by the metrics are listed in Table 1. The results on these 3 representative volumes further demonstrate the efficiency of the proposed method.

In practice, the proposed method performs poorly for tiny tumors with low contrast between the surrounded liver parenchyma and tumors on the low intensity liver parenchyma which are shown in Fig. 4.

The reasons of these failed segmentation can be attributed to the invalid feature extraction in the complex abdomen CT volumes. All these cases presented

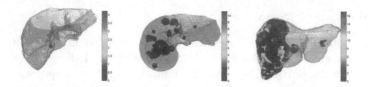

Fig. 3. Segmentation results of the proposed method. (a) no. 3 of LiTS, (b) no. 19. of 3D-IRCADb and (c) no. 4 of LiTS.

Table 1. Quantitative comparison results in Fig. 3

Volume	VOE	RVD	ASD	RMSD	MSD	Sensitivity	Specificity	Accuracy
(a)	0.17	0.47	0.84	1.10	3.64	0.93	0.97	0.98
(b)	0.13	1.40	0.96	1.78	9.96	0.94	0.96	0.95
(c)	1.04	1.23	0.76	2.25	15.03	0.97	0.99	0.99

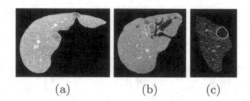

(a)   (b)   (c)

Fig. 4. Challenge of tumor segmentation in CT images.

are open challenge in tumor segmentation. Other failed segmentation comes from the missed liver mask location of FCN. We will research further to solve these problems in our future work.

4   Conclusion

In this study, we proposed a novel automatic method to isolate liver tumors from abdomen CT images. The proposed method makes full use of the advantage of FCN 3D to automatic localization and deformable model to refine surface. The deformable model is derived from NMF and driven by LCSH. Experimental results on clinical data demonstrated that the proposed segmentation method achieves satisfactory results. We concluded that the proposed method is a promising method for automatic tumors segmentation.

Acknowledgments. This research is sponsored by the National Natural Science Foundation of China (61472053, 91420102), Major Program of National Natural Science Foundation of China (No. 61190122), National Key Technology R&D Program of China (No. 2012BAI06B01).

References

1. Becker, M., Magnenat-Thalmann, N.: Deformable models in medical image segmentation. In: Magnenat-Thalmann, N., Ratib, O., Choi, H.F. (eds.) 3D Multiscale Physiological Human, pp. 81–106. Springer, London (2014). doi:10.1007/978-1-4471-6275-9_4
2. Chan, T.F., Esedoglu, S., Nikolova, M.: Algorithms for finding global minimizers of image segmentation and denoising models. SIAM J. Appl. Math. **66**(5), 1632–1648 (2006)
3. Chen, B., Chen, Y., Yang, G., Meng, J., Zeng, R., Luo, L.: Segmentation of liver tumor via nonlocal active contours. In: 2015 IEEE International Conference on Image Processing (ICIP), pp. 3745–3748. IEEE (2015)
4. Christ, P.F., et al.: Automatic liver and lesion segmentation in CT using cascaded fully convolutional neural networks and 3D conditional random fields. In: Ourselin, S., Joskowicz, L., Sabuncu, M.R., Unal, G., Wells, W. (eds.) MICCAI 2016. LNCS, vol. 9901, pp. 415–423. Springer, Cham (2016). doi:10.1007/978-3-319-46723-8_48
5. Gao, M., Chen, H., Zheng, S., Fang, B.: A factorization based active contour model for texture segmentation. In: 2016 IEEE International Conference on Image Processing (ICIP), pp. 4309–4313. IEEE (2016)
6. Göçeri, E.: Fully automated liver segmentation using sobolev gradient-based level set evolution. Int. J. Numeri. Methods Biomed. Eng. **32**(11) (2016)
7. Goldstein, T., Osher, S.: The split bregman method for l1-regularized problems. SIAM J. Imaging Sci. **2**(2), 323–343 (2009)
8. Götz, M., Heim, E., März, K., Norajitra, T., Hafezi, M., Fard, N., Mehrabi, A., Knoll, M., Weber, C., Maier-Hein, L., Maier-Hein, K.H.: A learning-based, fully automatic liver tumor segmentation pipeline based on sparsely annotated training data. In: Medical Imaging 2016: Image Processing (2016)
9. Heimann, T., Van Ginneken, B., Styner, M.A., Arzhaeva, Y., Aurich, V., Bauer, C., Beck, A., Becker, C., Beichel, R., Bekes, G.: Comparison and evaluation of methods for liver segmentation from CT datasets. IEEE Trans. Med. Imaging **28**(8), 1251–1265 (2009)
10. Krinidis, S., Chatzis, V.: A robust fuzzy local information C-means clustering algorithm. IEEE Trans. Image Process. **19**(5), 1328–1337 (2010)
11. Li, B.N., Chui, C.K., Chang, S., Ong, S.H.: A new unified level set method for semi-automatic liver tumor segmentation on contrast-enhanced CT images. Expert Syst. Appl. **39**(10), 9661–9668 (2012)
12. Patil, D.D., Deore, S.G.: Medical image segmentation: a review. Int. J. Comput. Sci. Mob. Comput. **2**(1), 22–27 (2013)
13. Shelhamer, E., Long, J., Darrell, T.: Fully convolutional networks for semantic segmentation. IEEE Trans. Pattern Anal. Mach. Intell. **39**(4), 640–651 (2017)
14. Shen, D., Wu, G., Suk, H.I.: Deep learning in medical image analysis. Ann. Rev. Biomed. Eng. **19**, 221–248 (2017)
15. Simonyan, K., Zisserman, A.: Very deep convolutional networks for large-scale image recognition. CoRR abs/1409.1556 (2014)
16. Yuan, J., Wang, D., Cheriyadat, A.M.: Factorization-based texture segmentation. IEEE Trans. Image Process. **24**(11), 3488–3497 (2015)
17. Zhang, K., Zhang, L., Lam, K.M., Zhang, D.: A level set approach to image segmentation with intensity inhomogeneity. IEEE Trans. Cybernet. **46**(2), 546–557 (2016)

Constructing Detailed Subject-Specific Models of the Human Masseter

C. Antonio Sánchez[1](✉), Zhi Li[2], Alan G. Hannam[3], Purang Abolmaesumi[1],
Anne Agur[2], and Sidney Fels[1]

[1] Department of Electrical and Computer Engineering,
University of British Columbia, Vancouver, BC, Canada
antonios@ece.ubc.ca

[2] Department of Surgery, University of Toronto, Toronto, ON, Canada

[3] Faculty of Dentistry, University of British Columbia, Vancouver, BC, Canada

Abstract. We investigate the structural details of the human masseter
and their contribution to force-transmission necessary for mastication
through a computational modelling study. We compare two subject-
specific models, constructed using data acquired by a dissection and
digitization procedure on cadaveric specimens. Despite architectural differences between the two masseters, we find that in both instances it is
necessary to capture the combination of the multipennate nature of the
muscle fibres, as well as the increased aponeurosis stiffness, in order to
reproduce adequate clenching forces. We also demonstrate the feasibility
of deformably registering these architectural templates to target muscle
surfaces in order to create new subject-specific models.

Keywords: Masseter · Mastication · Finite element · Aponeuroses

1 Introduction

Mastication, the chewing of food, is an important process that when hindered
can severely affect quality of life. In patients who have undergone treatment
for head and neck cancer, muscle damage due to either surgical resection or
radiotherapy often leads to reduced comminution efficiency, and can result in
chewing or swallowing disorders such as dysphagia. Understanding the mechanics
of mastication is crucial if we are to tailor interventions to subjects in order to
maximize post-treatment function.

Due to the complexity of the masticatory system, and that functional muscle
characteristics are difficult to isolate and measure without interfering with the
chewing cycle, computational biomechanical models have become indispensable
in studying the process. For simulations to be reliable, however, they must capture all relevant interactions of the coupled system of bones, tendons, muscles,
and other soft-tissues, as well as account for any subject-specific variability. To
this end, we are developing a detailed model of the masseter, the major muscle
involved in mastication, to study the impact of its structural characteristics on
function.

M.J. Cardoso et al. (Eds.): BIVPCS/POCUS 2017, LNCS 10549, pp. 52–60, 2017.
DOI: 10.1007/978-3-319-67552-7_7

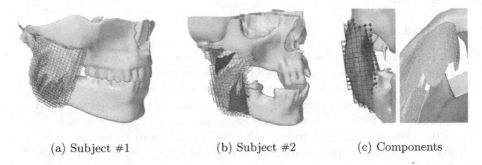

(a) Subject #1   (b) Subject #2   (c) Components

Fig. 1. Finite-element models of the masseter and jaw for simulating clenching force during mastication. The models consist of encapsulating hexahedral muscle volumes, attached to the mandible and zygomatic arch (blue nodes in (c)-left), which are coupled to thin interior membrane-like aponeuroses ((c)-right). (Color figure online)

Most existing models of mastication rely on line-based, lumped-parameter muscle models. Tanaka et al. [15] apply line-based models of the masseter acting on a finite element model (FEM) of the mandible to study stress distributions during teeth clenching. To study the dynamics of jaw-gaping, Hannam et al. [4] developed a complete jaw-hyoid model with line-based muscles. Stavness et al. [14] later used this model to predict muscle activations and forces required for chewing. These line-based representations of the masseter are somewhat limited: they assume muscle uniformity, cannot represent broad attachment areas, and cannot be used to predict stresses within the muscle volume. To examine the impact of surgical intervention or treatment on muscle function, we need a more-detailed three-dimensional representation of the structure.

To our knowledge, Röhrle et al. [12] created the only existing finite-element model of the masseter. They show that using line-based muscles can introduce significant errors in simulated force distributions, to the point where different clinical outcomes could be predicted. One of the limitations of the study was a low prediction of maximum bite force: 77 N, which is quite shy of the potential 200 N+ which has been observed in practice [7]. They note that muscle fibre distribution plays an important role, and suggest that the model can be improved by including a more accurate representation of the muscle architecture.

Unfortunately, the internal details of the masseter are extremely challenging to see using conventional imaging techniques [11]. Because of this, we have acquired two uniquely detailed architectural descriptions of the masseter through dissection and digitization studies. In this work we describe our process for incorporating this data into an efficient hybrid simulation model, which will later be included in a larger complete model for studying mastication.

2   Methods

2.1   Data Collection

Data used for modelling was collected from two human cadaveric studies using the dissection and digitization procedure of Kim et al. [6] (Fig. 2). In this procedure, the formalin embalmed tissue was exposed by removing any skin and superficial fascia. The specimens were securely clamped, and three screws afixed to the bone to act as a frame of reference. The muscle surface was cleaned and delineated to allow each muscle fibre bundle (fascicle) to be traced in its entirety. Digitization of muscle fascicles was carried out using a MicroScribe™ MX Digitizer (0.05 mm accuracy; Immersion Corporation, San Jose, CA). Each fascicle was traced at 3–5 mm intervals between attachment sites. The fibres were then excised to reveal underlying fascicles and aponeuroses. The dissection and digitization process continued until the entire muscle volume was captured. Ethics approval for this study was received from University of Toronto Health Sciences, Mount Sinai Hospital, and University of British Columbia Research Ethics Boards (P.R. #27210, #28530, 12-0252-E, H12-00130).

The first data set, described in Leon et al. [9], was initially collected to study fibre motions during opening and closing of the jaw. Unfortunately, no information regarding aponeuroses was acquired, so for our modelling efforts they were manually drawn based on terminating fibre ends and from anatomical references. For the second specimen, it was decided to additionally digitize the aponeuroses, beginning with the perimeter, then following collagen fibre bundles on the exposed surface. To form three-dimensional sheets of aponeuroses, these outlines were transformed into NURBS curves using Autodesk Maya® and surfaces were lofted between them. A CT scan of the second specimen was also acquired (Aquilion ONE™, Toshiba Medical Systems Corporation, Tokyo, Japan) with resolution 2 mm × 2 mm and slice thickness of 3 mm. The skull was segmented using thresholding, and manually aligned with the digitized muscle data.

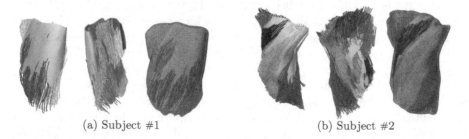

(a) Subject #1   (b) Subject #2

Fig. 2. Digitized muscle fascicles, internal aponeuroses, and encapsulating muscle volume for two subjects. Colours reflect distinct groups of muscle fascicles.

2.2   Finite Element Model Construction

To build volumetric muscle models from the digitized data, we first need to create an encapsulating muscle volume. Similar to Lee et al. [8], we constructed a wrapping surface around the collection of fibres and aponeuroses. For this, we start by computing a three-dimensional distance field on a $100 \times 80 \times 35$ grid of points, determining the distance of each grid point to the nearest 'feature' (either a line-segment from the digitized fibre bundles or face from the triangulated aponeurosis surfaces). We smooth the distance grid by applying the Laplacian smoothing operator, then reconstruct a continuous field by trilinearly interpolating between the grid points. To create the bounding surface, we extract an iso-surface from the smoothed field using the Marching Tetrahedra algorithm [3]. For our masseters, we chose the 2 mm iso-surface.

The next step is to construct the three-dimensional finite-element mesh. Due to the highly incompressible nature of muscle tissue, hexahedral elements are preferred as they avoid common volumetric locking artifacts exhibited by tetrahedral elements. Unfortunately, for our complex geometry including the thin aponeuroses, constructing conforming hexahedral meshes is an extremely challenging and labour-intensive task. Instead, we follow Teran et al. [16], and create a non-conforming bounding finite-element mesh of the entire muscle volume. The result is a voxelized representation, consisting of 1419 and 969 linear 8-node hexahedral elements for the two models (Fig. 1). The muscle-specific material law requires determining the fibre orientation at each point of numerical integration within the FEM volume. We define a fibre field for each compartment of digitized fibre bundles using the method of Sánchez et al. [13]: around each integration point, we examine an influence radius ($r = 2$ mm), and compute a weighted average orientation of all contained digitized fibre segments. These orientations then define the directions of muscle contraction within the corresponding elements.

For the aponeuroses, we extrude the triangulated surface meshes to create 0.5 mm-thin wedge elements. We detach the top nodes of neighbouring elements in order to mimic a membrane, which exhibits in-plane elastic behaviour but zero bending stiffness (Fig. 1c). This allows the aponeuroses to perform their function of transmitting forces to the muscle attachment sites without overly stiffening the entire muscle volume. We then couple the bounding hexahedral FEM and membrane-like aponeurotic sheets using a system of constraints. For each node that falls on the original aponeurosis surface, we compute the values of the FEM interpolation functions $\{\phi_j(t)\}$ at rest such that

$$t_i^{(0)} = \sum_j \phi_j\left(t_i^{(0)}\right) m_j^{(0)}, \tag{1}$$

where $t_i^{(0)}$ is the location of the ith node on the aponeurotic sheets at time 0, and $m_j^{(0)}$ is the location of the jth node in the encapsulating muscle volume. To enforce coupling of the models, we maintain this relationship as time progresses, effectively binding the node to its barycentric coordinate within the corresponding muscle element. We can express the constraints as $\mathbf{G}n = 0$, where n is a concatenated vector of node positions including both muscle nodes m and tendon (aponeurosis) nodes t, and $\mathbf{G}$ is a constraint matrix consisting of the fixed interpolation coefficients from Eq. (1).

For our first masseter model (Fig. 1a), we manually aligned the masseter volume with Hannam's existing model for mastication [4] so that fibre bundle ends and aponeuroses aligned with the appropriate origin and insertion sites on the zygomatic arch and angle/ramus of the mandible. For the second model (Fig. 1b), we similarly manually registered the muscle to the skull and jaw extracted from CT. We then attached the muscle volumes to these rigid components by securing nodes to the bones based on proximity as in Fig. 1c.

2.3 Constitutive Laws

We model both the underlying muscle tissue and aponeuroses as incompressible Mooney-Rivlin hyperelastic solids with strain-energy density function

$$W(I_1, I_2, J) = c_1(I_1 - 3) + c_2(I_2 - 3) + \kappa(J - 1)^2, \tag{2}$$

where I_1 and I_2 are the first and second invariants of the Cauchy-Green deformation tensor, and J is the determinant of the deformation gradient. The constants c_1 and c_2 are stiffness parameters, and κ is the bulk modulus responsible for incompressibility. To include the anisotropic contraction behaviour of muscles, we add a material stress based on the Blemker [1] constitutive model:

$$\sigma(\lambda) = \sigma_{\max}\left(\alpha f_{\text{act}}(\lambda) + f_{\text{pass}}(\lambda)\right)(\lambda/\lambda_{\text{opt}}), \tag{3}$$

where $\sigma_{\max}$ is the maximum isometric stress in the muscle, $\alpha \in [0, 1]$ is the normalized muscle activation level, λ is the along-fibre stretch, λ_{opt} is the optimal fibre stretch, and f_{act} and f_{pass} are normalized functions that describe the active and passive force-length relationships for the muscle, respectively (see [1]). For our simulations, we use the same values as Röhrle et al., $c_1 = c_2 = 10$ kPa, $\sigma_{\max} = 300$ kPa, and $\lambda_{\text{opt}} = 1.4$. For the aponeurosis material, we increase c_1 and c_2 by a factor of 100 to represent its stiff tensile behaviour.

2.4 Simulation, Registration and Results

For our numerical simulations, we use the open-source ArtiSynth platform [10]. ArtiSynth allows us to combine rigid and deformable elements, along with constraints and coupling, in a hybrid simulation environment. We fix the location of the jaw and skull, activate the muscle, and measure the net isometric contraction force acting between the bones. We take this to be our clenching force contribution from each masseter.

To determine the impact of the various architectural properties, we ran three simulations for each model. In the first, we ignore all internal details, only using the muscle's outer shape with a simplified muscle fibre direction field acting between muscle origin and insertion sites, as in [12]. For the second simulation, we

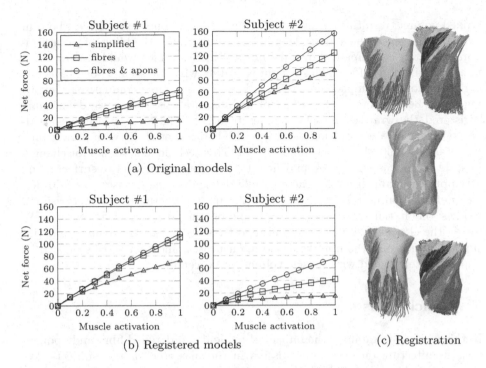

(a) Original models

(b) Registered models

(c) Registration

Fig. 3. Force production in the masseter during clenching, applied to both original and registered models. In (c), we see the original (top) and registered (bottom) muscle volumes. The volume from subject #1 (pink) was deformed to fit the muscle surface from subject #2 (cyan). This provides an architectural mapping between the two. (Color figure online)

replace the simplified field with the one derived from muscle fascicle digitization. For the third, we add our thin coupled aponeuroses models, including their stiff tension properties. Force results are shown in Fig. 3a.

In both subject-specific models, use of the simplified directional fibre field resulted in the lowest peak force (14 N, 96 N). Adding the detailed pennated fibre architecture significantly increases force (55 N, 125 N), and incorporating the aponeuroses increased force even further (64 N, 157 N). For subject #1, the aponeuroses did not have as strong an impact as for subject #2. This may be related to our uncertainty in reconstructing the aponeurotic sheets, since the fibre field was less dense and we had no measurements of the collagen fibres. The larger discrepancy between the two models, however, seems to be related to muscle volume. The estimated masseter volume for the first subject, based on the wrapped-fibre surface, is $19.7\,\text{cm}^3$, whereas for the second subject is $38.8\,\text{cm}^3$.

The most reliable predictor of a muscle's peak force is its physiological cross-sectional area (PCSA), which is measured perpendicular to its fibres [8]. The muscle's architecture therefore plays a significant role: the fibre pennation and attachments to internal aponeuroses allow for a larger cross-sectional area within a fixed volume, resulting in the capacity for stronger contraction forces. For our two models, since the muscle lengths are similar, the doubling of volume is approximately accompanied by a doubling of PCSA, which would in-turn result in a doubling of net force. This is approximately what we seem to be observing.

To remove the impact of muscle volume on our force comparisons, allowing us to better examine the effect of architectural intricacies, we deformably registered the wrapped muscle volumes together (Fig. 3c). We use the FEM-based deformable registration technique of Khallaghi et al. [5] with parameters: $\beta = 1000$, $E = 60$ kPa, $\nu = 0.49$, $w = 0.05$. This technique accounts for changes in scale, estimates soft-correspondences between points on the two surfaces, and attempts to minimize strain energy while deforming one dataset to the other. The deformation map is invertible, allowing us to construct two new registered models: one in the space of subject #1, and one in the space of subject #2. We re-ran the clenching simulations, and report results in Fig. 3b. Again, we notice similar influence of the fibre field and aponeuroses, and that force seems to be approximately scaled with muscle volume as expected.

3   Conclusions

In this work, we examined the impact of modelling a detailed fibre and aponeurosis architecture on force transmission in the masseter for two subjects. We showed that by including both the pennated fibre field and the stiff aponeurotic sheets, we were able to increase simulated maximum bite forces to more realistic levels in subject #2 (167 N *vs.* 96 N). In subject #1, we also saw gains in force, but the values themselves were much smaller. We hypothesize that we are currently under-representing the muscle volume for this subject, which seems to be confirmed by registering the model to the muscle volume of subject #2. This resulted in an increased maximum net force from 64 N to 157 N.

The dissection process clearly cannot be used to extract architectural details in live subjects. Instead, we propose to register our current digitized templates to muscle surfaces extracted by other means such as image segmentation. We demonstrated the feasibility of this approach by registering our two masseters together to create two new registered models. The force patterns in the registered models are on similar orders of magnitude as their target counterparts, but still do exhibit differences. This suggests that a significant portion of force-production can be accounted-for by adjusting for muscle shape and volume, but that subject-specific architectural variability may still play an important role. With new advanced imaging techniques (e.g. [2]), we may be able to obtain some of these internal muscle details *in vivo*. We could then combine this data with our template-based approach, using it for both for template selection and for adding internal targets during registration. Such a hybrid technique would allow us to quickly and efficiently generate subject-specific models of the masseter for studying and analyzing the functional impact of treatment on mastication.

Acknowledgments. This work was supported by the Natural Sciences and Engineering Research Council of Canada (NSERC), the Canadian Institutes of Health Research (CIHR), and the University of British Columbia.

References

1. Blemker, S., Pinsky, P., Delp, S.: A 3D model of muscle reveals the causes of nonuniform strains in the biceps brachii. J. Biomech. **38**(4), 657–665 (2005)
2. Cioffi, I., Gallo, L.M., Palla, S., Erni, S., Farella, M.: Macroscopic analysis of human masseter compartments assessed by magnetic resonance imaging. Cells Tissues Organs **195**(5), 465–472 (2012)
3. Doi, A., Koide, A.: An efficient method of triangulating equi-valued surfaces by using tetrahedral cells. IEICE Trans. Inf. Syst. **74**(1), 214–224 (1991)
4. Hannam, A., Stavness, I., Lloyd, J., Fels, S.: A dynamic model of jaw and hyoid biomechanics during chewing. J. Biomech. **41**(5), 1069–1076 (2008)
5. Khallaghi, S., Sánchez, C.A., Rasoulian, A., Nouranian, S., Romagnoli, C., Abdi, H., Chang, S.D., Black, P.C., Goldenberg, L., Morris, W.J., Spadinger, I., Fenster, A., Ward, A., Fels, S., Abolmaesumi, P.: Statistical biomechanical surface registration: application to MR-TRUS fusion for prostate interventions. IEEE Trans. Med. Imaging **34**(12), 2535–2549 (2015)
6. Kim, S.Y., Boynton, E.L., Ravichandiran, K., Fung, L.Y., Bleakney, R., Agur, A.M.: Three-dimensional study of the musculotendinous architecture of supraspinatus and its functional correlations. Clin. Anat. **20**(6), 648–655 (2007)
7. Koolstra, J., van Eijden, T., Weijs, W., Naeije, M.: A three-dimensional mathematical model of the human masticatory system predicting maximum possible bite forces. J. Biomech. **21**(7), 563–576 (1988)
8. Lee, D., Ravichandiran, K., Jackson, K., Fiume, E., Agur, A.: Robust estimation of physiological cross-sectional area and geometric reconstruction for human skeletal muscle. J. Biomech. **45**(8), 1507–1513 (2012)
9. Leon, L.M., Liebgott, B., Agur, A.M., Norwich, K.H.: Computational model of the movement of the human muscles of mastication during opening and closing of the jaw. CMBBE **9**(6), 387–398 (2006)
10. Lloyd, J.E., Stavness, I., Fels, S.: ArtiSynth: a fast interactive biomechanical modeling toolkit combining multibody and finite element simulation. In: Payan, Y. (ed.) Soft Tissue Biomechanical Modeling for Computer Assisted Surgery. Studies in Mechanobiology, Tissue Engineering and Biomaterials, vol. 11, pp. 355–394. Springer, Heidelberg (2012). doi:10.1007/8415_2012_126
11. Raadsheer, M., van Eijden, T., van Spronsen, P., van Ginkel, F., Kiliaridis, S., Prahl-Andersen, B.: A comparison of human masseter muscle thickness measured by ultrasonography and magnetic resonance imaging. Arch. Oral Biol. **39**(12), 1079–1084 (1994)
12. Röhrle, O., Pullan, A.J.: Three-dimensional finite element modelling of muscle forces during mastication. J. Biomech. **40**(15), 3363–3372 (2007)
13. Sánchez, C.A., Lloyd, J.E., Fels, S., Abolmaesumi, P.: Embedding digitized fibre fields in finite element models of muscles. Comput. Methods Biomech. Biomed. Eng. Imaging Vis. **1**(4) (2013)
14. Stavness, I., Hannam, A.G., Lloyd, J.E., Fels, S.: Predicting muscle patterns for hemimandibulectomy models. CMBBE **13**(4), 483–491 (2010)

15. Tanaka, E., Tanne, K., Sakuda, M.: A three-dimensional finite element model of the mandible including the tmj and its application to stress analysis in the tmj during clenching. Med. Eng. Phys. **16**(4), 316–322 (1994)

16. Teran, J., Sifakis, E., Blemker, S., Ng-Thow-Hing, V., Lau, C., Fedkiw, R.: Creating and simulating skeletal muscle from the visible human data set. IEEE Trans. Vis. Comput. Graph. **11**(3), 317–328 (2005)

MRI-Based Heart and Torso Personalization for Computer Modeling and Simulation of Cardiac Electrophysiology

Ernesto Zacur[1]([✉]), Ana Minchole[2], Benjamin Villard[1], Valentina Carapella[4], Rina Ariga[3], Blanca Rodriguez[2], and Vicente Grau[1]

[1] Department of Engineering Science, Institute of Biomedical Engineering,
University of Oxford, Oxford, UK
ernesto.zacur@eng.ox.ac.uk
[2] Department of Computer Science, University of Oxford, Oxford, UK
[3] Division of Cardiovascular Medicine, University of Oxford Centre
for Clinical Magnetic Resonance Research, Oxford, UK
[4] Simula Research Laboratory, Bærum, Norway

Abstract. In the last decade, electrophysiological models for *in-silico* simulations of cardiac electrophysiology have gained much attention in the research field. However, to translate them to clinical uses, the models need personalization based on recordings from the patient. In this work, we explore methodologies for the patient-specific personalization of torso and heart geometric models based on standard clinical cardiac magnetic resonance acquisitions to enable simulations. The inclusion of the torso and its internal structures allows simulations of the human ventricular electrophysiological activity from the ionic level to the body surface potentials and to the electrocardiogram.

1 Introduction

Biophysical electrophysiological (EP) models for the simulation of the electrical activity of the human heart are now approaching a mature state and are ready to be translated from an academic setting to medical research and clinical environments. Multiscale human ventricular EP models encapsulate mechanisms at the ionic and cellular level and incorporate a representation of tissue coupling to describe the propagation of the electrical excitation up to the whole organ (heart) electrical activity. *In-silico* simulations of virtual hearts present a research framework for the interpretation of medical data, allowing the assessment of biological hypothesis. In addition, they can be used to predict outcomes under simulated conditions such as cardiac or physiological dysfunctions, remodeling of the cardiac tissue, or drug treatments. Recently, EP models have moved from the study of general templates, either from a single subject or synthetic geometries, to be used with patient personalized data. This will be extended in the near future to play a role in the clinic to understand pathologies, stratify diseases, and also to optimize therapies. Several works have already made progress towards patient-specific personalized modeling, for example [1, 2]. Structural and functional information of the heart

© Springer International Publishing AG 2017
M.J. Cardoso et al. (Eds.): BIVPCS/POCUS 2017, LNCS 10549, pp. 61–70, 2017.
DOI: 10.1007/978-3-319-67552-7_8

is a key aspect in the personalization of the model. Patient-specific characteristics of the anatomy of the heart can be included into EP models by means of imaging studies including computer tomography (CT), magnetic resonance imaging, or ultrasound techniques. In particular, cardiac magnetic resonance (CMR) techniques provide a broad anatomical and functional information in a non-invasive manner and have become a routine diagnostic tool for some cardiovascular diseases. However, clinical CMR studies tend to consist of a sparse set of independent slices, which makes three-dimensional representation challenging.

Patient-specific electrical activities of the heart can be directly measured. Endocardial mappings record electrical signals by placing an electrode in different positions of the left endocardium using a catheter, and epicardial mappings get direct measures at the epicardial surface in an open chest surgery. Besides those invasive measures, body surface potential (BSP) mapping and the routinely used in the clinic electrocardiogram (ECG) measure the electrical activity of the heart non-invasively but in an indirect and global way.

In this work, we present a CMR based technique to geometrically personalize *in-silico* human cardiac models from patient's CMR to enable forward EP simulations from the ionic level to the BSPs. The inclusion of the torso enables specifically the simulation of the electrocardiogram, which is the most widely used tool for evaluation of the human heart activity. It is worth mentioning that our proposed anatomical personalization could also be used in an inverse problem setting going from measured BSPs to epicardial activity. We will show that it is possible to accurately reconstruct the bi-ventricular and torso anatomy of the patient from a standard CMR acquisition protocol used in clinical practice with no more than *localizers* (scout images acquired at the beginning of the CMR session), 4-chamber and 2-chamber views and a stack of short axis slices from the base to the apex of the left ventricle in cine acquisition. Using standard CMR protocols is an important point since acquisition time in the clinic is a very limited and demanding resource and more extensive acquisition protocols are generally relegated to research. The focus on magnetic resonance studies is motivated by its noninvasiveness and also because of the ability of CMR studies to characterize multiple structural and functional parameters including scars, tissue or fiber microstructure, fat deposits, infarcted or fibrotic areas.

2   Methods

This section presents the details of our patient-specific reconstruction of a heart-torso anatomy derived from clinical CMR images with the final purpose to be used in an EP simulation framework up to the BSPs. Sample results for each step are shown together with the explanation of the methods.

Bi-ventricular cardiac anatomy

The cardiac tissue is segmented from long axis (LAX) views (4- and 2-chambers views) as well as from the stack of short axis (SAX) views of a cine acquisition. There are several software tools to perform tissue segmentation, including commercial products widely used in the clinical practice (see [3] for references) as well as other research tools (for example, [4]). These offer different degrees of automation, from complete manual contouring, semiautomatic methods to reduce the operator time, up to fully automated tools. Which of them is the best option for cardiac images is debatable, on the one hand, manual contouring is usually considered as a ground truth, while automatic methods avoid operator bias, unintentional errors and have repeatability. In this work, we use manual contours from a well-trained expert with several years of experience. The contouring follows the general guidelines and consensus recommendations from [5]. Contouring includes left epicardium (including the septum), left endocardium (excluding papillary muscles), and right endocardium from and to the septum (excluding trabeculations). Exemplary LAX and SAX contours are shown in Fig. 1. Images in the example correspond to the end diastolic (ED) frame.

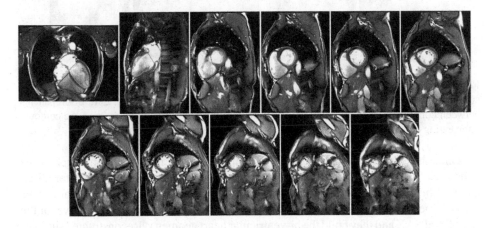

Fig. 1. Heart cine slices and their contours at ED. From left to right and from top to bottom: 4- and 2-chamber views, short axis stack from the most basal to the most apical slice. Left epicardium contours in red, left endocardium contours in green, and right endocardium contours in blue. (Color figure online)

Since we are interested in bi-ventricular geometry, the right ventricle endocardium borders are needed. However, the image resolution does not usually allow an accurate delineation. Therefore, we synthesize the right epicardium contour as an offset of the right endocardium at a distance of 4 mm [6]. After that, contours are automatically reorganized into a complete epicardial contour (EPI), the left endocardium (LV), and the right endocardium (RV), now including the septum (see Fig. 2).

Due to different cine slices being acquired at different breath holds, misalignments and spatial inconsistencies usually appear among the contours. We use the methodology described in [7] to correct for these misalignments. In summary, the alignment method computes the optimal rigid transformation in 3D for each slice for the contours to define spatially consistent surfaces. Realigned contours are shown in Fig. 3.

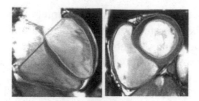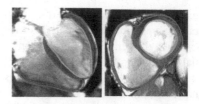

Fig. 2. Re-organization of the contours: synthesis of the right epicardium as part of the whole epicardium and split the left ventricle into epicardium and septum.

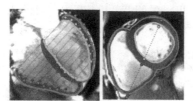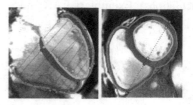

Fig. 3. Alignment of the slices to correct the breath motion. The spatial consistency of the contours is improved as can be seen in the lateral wall of the right ventricle. Left: discrepancies between contours from intersecting slices before correction. Right: after correction the contours intersecting contours are more consistent.

Once the contours are consistently aligned, a surface is interpolated for each of the structures (EPI, LV, and RV), following [8]. As in the case of the correction for alignment of the slices, the use of LAX views is key at this step. In particular, the apical area can only be well resolved using LAXs. The three surfaces are clipped at the level of the most basal SAX and they build the bi-ventricular heart geometry. Reconstructed surfaces together with the contours are shown in Fig. 4.

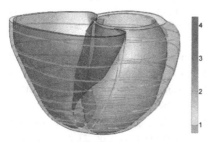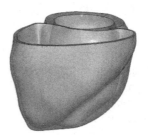

Fig. 4. Left: contours and the reconstructed surfaces of the heart. Each contour point is colored according to its distance to the corresponding surface (distances in mm). Right: another view of the final bi-ventricular heart.

Body and torso anatomy

Unlike CT, cine CMR does not usually produce a volumetric image but a sparse set of 3D oriented slices. Therefore classical surface generation techniques from volumetric data such as marching cubes cannot be used. This makes the reconstruction of the body surface (BS) challenging since only very sparse information of the torso is available. Some previous approaches have dealt with this scenario to reconstruct the body: [9] proposes a human model customization from monocular photos; [10] uses a manual affine deformation of a template to sagittal, coronal and axial MR images; [11] combined CT and MRI scans to make a tetrahedral mesh of a pig thorax; and [12] also uses MRI and CT scans to personalize a human geometry. In this work, we propose to fit a statistical shape model (SSM) of human bodies to the BS contours that we can obtain from the MR images. Although the CMR images are not acquired with a focus on body surface extraction, their field of view normally includes parts of the BS. Besides, at the start of the CMR studies, scout images in sagittal, coronal and axial views are commonly acquired to be used as localizers. We contoured the BS from all these images, using a semiautomatic tool that extracts isophote curves in the clearly contrasted interface between air and skin. The extracted contours are shown in Fig. 5, where the sparsity of the data can be appreciated as well as the presence of large regions (such as the upper-right part of the chest) with no information at all.

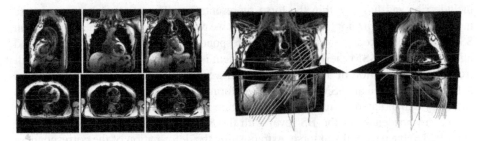

Fig. 5. Left: BS contours on the localizers. Right: 3D arrangement of all the BS controls, including the ones that can be extracted from heart focused slices (see Fig. 1).

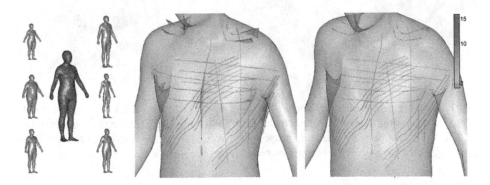

Fig. 6. Left: mean shape of the body SSM with its extreme shapes along the 1st, 2nd, and 3rd principal modes. Center: the result of the SSM fitted to the body contours. Points of the contours are colored according to their distances to the surface. Right: the result of TPS deformation towards the contour points to reduce the contour-to-surface distances.

A SSM of body shapes[1] built from 4300 subjects [13] is fitted to the contours. A rigid transformation together with the first 40 principal components of the SSM were considered in the fitting. As initial condition, the mean shape is situated in accordance with the previously reconstructed heart. The fitting is performed by a gradient descent to minimize the root mean square (RMS) contours-to-surface distance. Figure 6 shows an example of the fitting with a final RMS of 6.7 mm. After the SSM fitting, a final deformation is performed via approximate thin plate splines (TPS) [14, 15] to improve the agreement with the contours, resulting in a final RMS of 3.4 mm.

Ribs and lungs

In order to compute BSPs, the electrical potentials at the heart surface have to be propagated to the skin. In that path, the impedances of the different tissues between the epicardium and the skin have to be considered. The inclusion of the different organs for computational studies is controversial with some works reporting minor contributions of different organ impedances on BSP [16] and others reporting significant effects due to uncertainty in impedances [17]. Therefore, for potential sensitivity analysis, we include ribs and lungs within the torso representation. These internal structures are incorporated through template deformation. As we represent the BS by a deformed mean SSM mesh with fixed anatomical point correspondences, a representation of ribs and lung in that mean SSM mesh coordinates system is sufficient. This template was built from the segmentation of a CT acquisition of a single subject, for which its BS was deformed to the mean SSM shape. The deformation of the internal structures was smoothly extrapolated by means of TPS. Figure 7 shows the ribs and lungs template with correspondences at the BS level with the SSM model. This template is finally deformed to the personalized torso, extrapolating the deformation of the correspondént anatomical points by TPS.

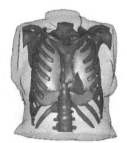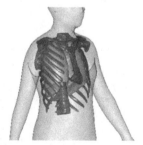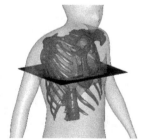

Fig. 7. Left: segmented internal structures of the torso obtained from a CT of a single subject. Center: transfer of the internal structures to the mean SSM shape. Left: deformation from the mean SSM to the patient personalized body shape (only ribs and lungs are transferred to the patient geometry whilst the heart is the one reconstructed from the patient images).

---

[1] http://humanshape.mpi-inf.mpg.de/.

Remeshing final surfaces and volumetric meshes
The majority of biophysical EP models are solved using the finite element method (FEM) with unstructured meshes of tetrahedral elements. The meshes allow the tessellation of complex geometric objects and the specification of different properties for each element depending on which structure it belongs to. In our case of a full body simulation, different spatial scales have to be considered. Spatial resolutions smaller than 0.5 mm are required to resolve the propagation of the electrical activation within the myocardium with acceptable accuracy. For example, a spatial resolution of 0.4 mm has been used in [18] to get an error in the conduction velocity below 10%. However, due to the different nature of the physical mechanism, larger spatial resolutions can be used to solve the propagation of the epicardial potentials to the BS. The heart surface (Fig. 4 right) is remeshed with a restricted Frontal-Delaunay algorithm using the mesh generator JIGSAW[2] [19] with a specified element size of 0.4 mm. The other structures are remeshed with the same software with the following element sizes: 2 mm for the ribs; 3 mm for the lungs; and 10 mm for the torso. Once surfaces have been remeshed, TETGEN[3] [20] is used to build the final tetrahedral mesh (see Fig. 9 left). The resulting tetrahedral meshes have a number of elements in the order of 40×10^6 (7×10^6 nodes), of which 30×10^6 (5×10^6 nodes) correspond to the myocardium.

3   Results

Figure 8 shows the acquired slices together with their intersection with the BS, ribs, and lungs for a visual assessment of the fitting of the torso and the placement of the internal structures. A quantitative assessment was performed in terms of the distances from the manual contour points to the reconstructed meshes. For the epicardium surface, the resulting RMS of contours-to-mesh distance is 0.5 mm with 90% of the points with a distance below to 0.75 mm. For the left endocardium, RMS is 1.35 mm and 90% percentile 2.2 mm. For the right endocardium, RMS is 0.45 mm and 90% percentile 0.72 mm. Finally, to evaluate the reconstruction of the body surface, RMS is 3.44 mm and 90% percentile 5.5 mm.

A bi-domain EP simulation following the O'Hara-Rudy model was conducted in CHASTE[4] [21] using the patient-specific personalized mesh. Early activation sites in the endocardium were selected in accordance with physiological knowledge [22]. Others physiological parameters were set to standard values found in the literature. Fiber microstructure was built following the Streeter rule from $-60°$ helix angle at endocardial surfaces to $+60°$ at epicardium [23]. BSPs were computed by propagating the electrical activity from the epicardium. Figure 9 depicts the obtained BSPs. In addition, we can virtually place electrodes on the limbs and the surface chest to synthesize a 12-lead ECG.

---

[2] http://github.com/dengwirda/jigsaw.
[3] http://wias-berlin.de/software/tetgen/.
[4] http://www.cs.ox.ac.uk/chaste/.

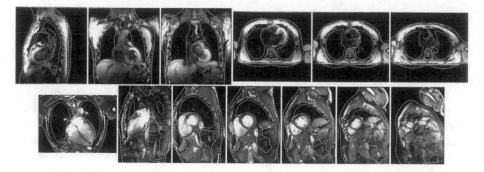

Fig. 8. Visual assessment of the fitted torso and the reconstructed internal surfaces. Dotted lines correspond to the manual delineations of the BS and continuous lines correspond to the intersection of the image plane with reconstructed the surfaces.

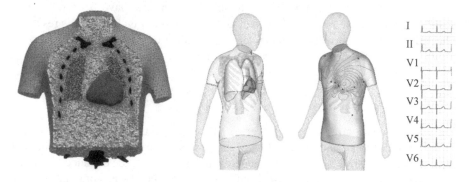

Fig. 9. From left to right: final tetrahedral mesh for FEM simulations (each internal structure having a label and specific properties); epicardial potentials (in arbitrary units) during the activation; isolevels of the BSPs and positions of the virtual electrodes (blue dots); synthesized ECG. (Color figure online)

4   Conclusion

We have described the components of a pipeline for the reconstruction of accurate patient-specific personalized models of heart and torso from CMR data. We show that model personalization can be performed using classical CMR protocols, with no need of extra acquisitions. The reconstruction of the torso geometry, with the accurate localization of the heart, allows the EP models to simulate the cardiac electrical activity from ionic currents up to the BS and the ECG. The inclusion of other structural and functional information from other CMR modalities such as scars or fibrotic areas can be easily performed. BSPs can be used to synthesize ECG signals that can be compared with the patient ECG. This pushes the use of *in-silico* EP models towards the clinical practice with several applications such as the understanding of pathologies, risk stratification, optimization and following of therapies.

Acknowledgments. EZ acknowledges the Marie Sklodowska-Curie Individual Fellowship from the H2020 EU Framework Programme for Research and Innovation (Proposal No: 655020-DTI4micro-MSCA-IF-EF-ST). AM and BR are supported by BR's Wellcome Trust Senior Research Fellowship in Basic Biomedical Sciences, the CompBiomed project (grant agreement No 675451) and the NC3R Infrastructure for Impact award (NC/P001076/1). BV acknowledges the support of the RCUK Digital Economy Programme grant number EP/G036861/1 (Oxford Centre for Doctoral Training in Healthcare Innovation). VC was supported by ERACoSysMed through a grant to the project SysAFib - Systems medicine for diagnosis and stratification of atrial fibrillation. RA is supported by a British Heart Foundation Clinical Research Training Fellowship. VG is supported by a BBSRC grant (BB/I012117/1), an EPSRC grant (EP/J013250/1), by BHF New Horizon Grant NH/13/30238 and by the CompBiomed project (grant agreement No 675451).

References

1. Arevalo, H., et al.: Arrhythmia risk stratification of patients after myocardial infarction using personalized heart models. Nature Commun. **7**, 11437 (2016)
2. Zettinig, O., et al.: From medical images to fast computational models of heart electromechanics: an integrated framework towards clinical use. In: Ourselin, S., Rueckert, D., Smith, N. (eds.) FIMH 2013. LNCS, vol. 7945, pp. 249–258. Springer, Heidelberg (2013). doi:10.1007/978-3-642-38899-6_30
3. Peng, P., et al.: A review of heart chamber segmentation for structural and functional analysis using cardiac MRI. Magn. Reson. Mater. Phys. **29**(2), 155–195 (2016)
4. Heiberg, E., et al.: Design and validation of segment - freely available software for cardiovascular image analysis. BMC Med. Imaging **10**(1), 1 (2010)
5. Schulz-Menger, J., et al.: Standardized image interpretation and post processing in cardiovascular magnetic resonance: Society for cardiovascular magnetic resonance (SCMR) board of trustees task force on standardized post processing. J. Cardiovasc. Magn. Reson. **15**(1), 35 (2013)
6. Prakash, R.: Determination of right ventricular wall thickness in systole and diastole. Echocardiographic and necropsy correlation in 32 patients. Heart **40**(11), 1257–1261 (1978)
7. Villard, B., Zacur, E., Dall'Armellina, E., Grau, V.: Correction of slice misalignment in multi-breath-hold cardiac MRI scans. In: Mansi, T., McLeod, K., Pop, M., Rhode, K., Sermesant, M., Young, A. (eds.) STACOM 2016. LNCS, vol. 10124, pp. 30–38. Springer, Cham (2017). doi:10.1007/978-3-319-52718-5_4
8. Villard, B., et al.: Cardiac mesh reconstruction from sparse, heterogeneous contours. In: Valdés Hernández, M., González-Castro, V. (eds.) MIUA 2017. CCIS, vol. 723, pp. 169–181. Springer, Cham (2017)
9. Zhu, S., et al.: An efficient human model customization method based on orthogonal view monocular photos. Comput. Aided Des. **45**(11), 1314–1332 (2013)
10. Zettinig, O., et al.: Data-driven estimation of cardiac electrical diffusivity from 12-lead ECG signals. Med. Image Anal. **18**(8), 1361–1376 (2014)
11. Gillette, K., et al.: Generation of combined-modality tetrahedral meshes. In: Proceedings CinC 2015 (2015)
12. Trayanova, N., et al.: How computer simulations of the human heart can improve anti-arrhythmia therapy. J. Physiol. **594**(9), 2483–2502 (2016)
13. Pishchulin, L., et al.: Building statistical shape spaces for 3D human modeling. Pattern Recogn. **67**, 276–286 (2017)

14. Rohr, K., et al.: Landmark-based elastic registration using approximating thin-plate splines. IEEE Trans. Med. Imaging **20**(6), 526–534 (2001)
15. Amberg, B., et al.: Optimal step nonrigid ICP algorithms for surface registration. In: Proceedings IEEE CVPR 2007 (2007)
16. Geneser, S., et al.: Application of stochastic FEM to study the sensitivity of ECG forward modeling to organ conductivity. IEEE Trans. Biomed. Eng. **55**(1), 31–40 (2008)
17. Keller, D., et al.: Ranking the influence of tissue conductivities on forward-calculated ECGs. IEEE Trans. Biomed. Eng. **57**(7), 1568–1576 (2010)
18. Bernabeu, M., et al.: Shock-induced arrhythmogenesis in the human heart: a computational modelling study. In: Proceedings IEEE EMBS 2010 (2010)
19. Engwirda, D.: Locally-optimal Delaunay-refinement and optimisation-based mesh generation. Ph.D. thesis, The University of Sydney (2014)
20. Hang, S.: TetGen, a Delaunay-based quality tetrahedral mesh generator. ACM Trans. Math. Softw. **41**(2), 11:1–11:36 (2015)
21. Pitt-Francis, J., et al.: Chaste: a test-driven approach to software development for biological modelling. Comput. Phys. Commun. **180**(12), 2452–2471 (2009)
22. Cardone-Noott, L., et al.: Human ventricular activation sequence and the simulation of the electrocardiographic QRS complex and its variability in healthy and intraventricular block conditions. EP Europace **18**(suppl. 4), iv4–iv15 (2016)
23. Streeter, D.: Gross Morphology and Fiber Geometry of the Heart. Johns Hopkins Press, Baltimore (1979)

Rapid Prediction of Personalised Muscle Mechanics: Integration with Diffusion Tensor Imaging

J. Fernandez[1,2(✉)], K. Mithraratne[1], M. Alipour[1], G. Handsfield[1],
T. Besier[1,2], and J. Zhang[1]

[1] Auckland Bioengineering Institute, University of Auckland, Auckland, New Zealand
j.fernandez@auckland.ac.nz
[2] Department of Engineering Science, University of Auckland, Auckland, New Zealand

Abstract. Diffusion Tensor Imaging (DTI) has been widely used to characterise the 3D fibre architecture in both neural and muscle mechanics. However, the computational expense associated with continuum models make their use in graphics and medical visualisation intractable. This study presents an integration of continuum muscle mechanics with partial least squares regression to create a fast mechano-statistical model. We use the human triceps surae muscle as an example informed though DTI. Our statistical models predicted muscle shape (within 0.063 mm RMS error), musculotendon force (within 1% error), and tissue strain (within 8% max error during contraction). Importantly, the presented framework may play a role in addressing computational cost of predicting detailed muscle information through popular rigid body solvers such as OpenSIM.

Keywords: Finite elements · Triceps surae muscle mechanics · Diffusion Tensor Imaging · Partial Least Squares Regression

1 Introduction

Muscle shape, stress, strain and overall function are strongly dictated by the underlying fibrous architecture. Muscle contraction along fibre paths determines how muscle interacts with the surrounding muscles and transfers loads to bone. The importance of anatomically accurate fibre descriptions for understanding muscle function was showcased by Nielsen et al. [1] who dissected a canine heart and digitised the 3D fibrous structure. The fibre information was fitted to a finite element field and used to simulate heart contraction [2, 3] amongst other applications. Lemos et al. [4] digitised cross-sectional images of a cat hind-limb to create a finite elastic model of the cat medial gastrocnemius, which described fibre orientation using 12 fibre bundles. Agur et al. [5] used cadaver tissue to build a 3D model of individual muscle fibre bundles in the human soleus. Around 400 individual bundles were fitted to a finite element field using B-Splines.

The use of DTI for skeletal muscle has become increasingly popular for identification of pennation angles and muscle function, however, its influence on 3D continuum mechanics simulations dictating contractile shape and deformation has received less attention. Muscle contraction using finite element analysis relies on correctly prescribing

© Springer International Publishing AG 2017
M.J. Cardoso et al. (Eds.): BIVPCS/POCUS 2017, LNCS 10549, pp. 71–77, 2017.
DOI: 10.1007/978-3-319-67552-7_9

the spatially varying fascicular orientation. This will have implications for moment arms in biomechanics, bone remodelling in orthopaedics and medical visualisation. One of the challenges in using continuum level muscle models is computational cost. Despite increases in high performance computing, complex finite element models are limited to small subject numbers. In order to translate computational tools to medical applications and large-scale visualisation we need to adopt population-based models. This concept uses the fact that large sets of pre-computed or measured data can be used to train a model using machine learning. This idea has been previously demonstrated including development of a surrogate knee model to predict joint contact [6], prediction of human femur cortical shell thickness [7], and lower limb shape prediction from a few sparse landmarks [8].

In this study we present a novel coupling between continuum mechanics simulations (demonstrated for the human triceps surae) and statistical methods. We report accuracy associated with rapid prediction of muscle force, shape and strain.

2   Methods

2.1   Geometry

Magnetic Resonance Imaging (MRI) was performed on the lower limb of a healthy subject using a T1–weighted spin echo sequence (Echo Time of 60 ms, Repeat Time of 4400 ms, NEX of 2 and size $2 \times 0.9 \times 0.9$ mm). The triceps surae muscles (gastrocnemius heads and soleus) were identified and manually digitised. In the same session a Diffusion Tensor Imaging (DTI) sequence was also performed. This allowed the two datasets to be easily registered. The limb was imaged from 20 different diffusion directions plus one baseline image.

Muscles fibres were determined using the Stejskal-Tanner equation [9], which relates the signal intensity without diffusion weighting, S_0, to the signal intensity with diffusion weighting in the kth direction, S_k, and is given by Eq. 1,

$$S_k = S_0 e^{-b\hat{g}_k^T D \hat{g}_k} \tag{1}$$

where, g_k, are the normalised diffusion gradient directions with k a minimum of 6 but typically being 20 or higher. D is the diffusion tensor and b is a factor controlling the amount of tissue diffusion allowed. For a standard MRI b is 0 (no diffusion), brain tissue typically uses 1000 and for the skeletal muscle tissue in this study we have used 500. By solving this equation system for each voxel in the volume image we can compute the diffusion tensor at each voxel, D. We used 20 directions (plus the references image with no diffusion) to compute the diffusion tensor, even though only 6 are necessary (assuming a symmetric tensor). This produced a 3×3 diffusion tensor for each voxel in the image volume, which was further diagonalised into 3 eigenvectors and eigenvalues. The underlying assumption is that the dominant eigenvector (which has the largest eigenvalue) is the main direction for fluid migration and aligned with the fibre direction in muscles. Each voxel will therefore produce a vector in the dominant direction, which when using tractography will provide a mapping of fibre information.

In order to estimate the errors in our DTI modelling pipeline we conducted a test using a simple phantom made from celery. Celery has been used frequently to evaluate DTI sequences given it has a strong parallel fibre orientation along its length. Eight celery sticks were placed in water and tightly sealed using a plastic container. Care was taken to ensure that no air pockets were present near the celery that can lead to artifacts in the DTI sequence. The celery fibres were then reconstructed using our presented pipeline and compared with the ideal digitised fibres.

Figure 1(left) shows the extracted fibre directions. This was fitted to a triceps surae finite element model using high-order cubic Hermite basis functions [10] shown in Fig. 1(middle). The muscle model presented here also forms part of a suite of musculoskeletal data within the International Union of Physiological Sciences (IUPS) Physiome Project repository [11], which is a framework for creation, sharing and dissemination of mathematical models of human physiology.

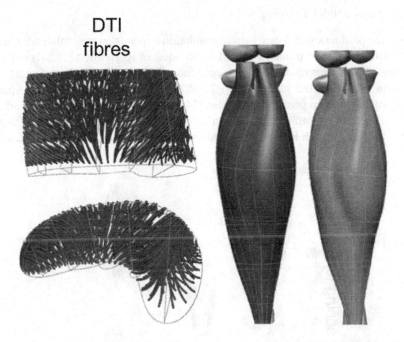

Fig. 1. (Left) Fitted DTI fibres from plan and cross-section view. (Middle) Undeformed triceps surae (red muscle). (Right) isometric contraction in gold. (Color figure online)

The fitted fibre field is used to inform a finite elastic mechanics contraction of muscle. For muscle we adopted a micro-structurally based constitutive law, the 'pole-zero' law [12] for passive muscle,

$$w = k_{\alpha\beta} \frac{E_{\alpha\beta}^2}{\left| a_{\alpha\beta} - E_{\alpha\beta} \right|^{b_{\alpha\beta}}} \tag{2}$$

where w is a strain energy density function, $E_{\alpha\beta}$ are Green's strain components referred to a DTI fibre axis, $a_{\alpha\beta}$ are the strain limits (poles) and $k_{\alpha\beta}$, $b_{\alpha\beta}$ are the scaling and curvature control parameters, respectively. The values used in this study are adapted from Fernandez and Hunter [12]. All values of $a_{\alpha\beta}$ and $b_{\alpha\beta}$ have been set to 1.0. The scaling coefficients were defined $k_{11} = 0.427$ MPa; $k_{22} = 0.1$ MPa and $k_{33} = 0.1$ MPa with the shear terms ($k_{\alpha\beta}$, $\alpha \neq \beta$) set to 0.001 MPa.

We simulated an isometric contraction for each muscle (constant length) using the HMT model of Hunter et al. [2]. Simulations were conducted by prescribing an incremental loading approach whereby the muscle activation was gradually increased to 800 N of muscle force (as seen during contralateral toe-off during gait [13]). The resulting muscle shape due to active contraction is highlighted as a gold muscle in Fig. 1(right).

2.2 Statistical Model Training

Muscle force production in a quasi-static simulation depends on musculotendon length and activation level. We trained a Partial Least Squares Regression (PLSR) model by simulating 36 scenarios (6 different musculotendon lengths for 6 different contraction states) from FE predicted models (Fig. 2). PLSR creates a linear model to predict response variables from predictor variables [14]. In this study, the predictor variables are musculotendon length and activation level, and the response variables are FE predicted muscle force, deformed shape and tissue strain. Model accuracy was assessed

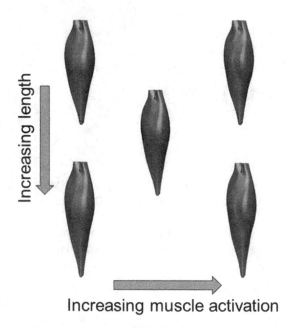

Fig. 2. Training the Partial Least Squares Regression model on 36 finite element triceps soleus simulations of different musculotendon length and activation combinations.

by doing a 'leave-one-out' analysis. One simulation from 36 was left out of the PLSR model and predicted independently. This was repeated for each simulation to report an average error.

3   Results

For the FE simulation it was observed that the triceps surae contracted with a distinct crease between the medial and lateral heads. The muscle slightly contracted longitudinally with minimum lateral expansion. The medial head was elevated and larger compared to the lateral head. These contractile characteristics are consistent with anatomy and provide confidence in the FE model predictions. The angle between the ideal fibre directions and the DTI processed fibre vectors was ~3° using our DTI fibre phantom.

The PLSR model predicted musculo-tendon force within 1% of the mechanical simulation. Figure 3(left) shows an example of muscle shape for 80% muscle stretch and maximum contraction. Blue is the FE mechanics simulation and red is the statistical prediction. All features of shape were predicted within a 0.063 mm RMS error. Figure 3 right shows the predicted largest principal component of strain. The principal components of strain as expected were aligned with the fibre directions. All strain vector fields were consistent between the mechanics and statistical model, however, the peak regions of strain magnitude were not predicted as well. The maximum error was within 8% between the mechanical and statistical model. This error was lower for smaller contractions.

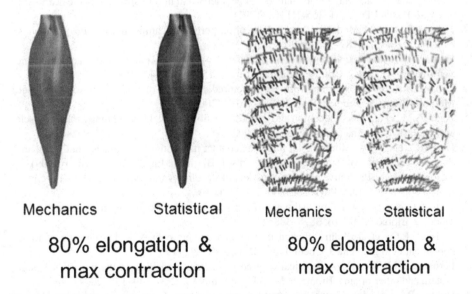

Mechanics   Statistical   Mechanics   Statistical

80% elongation & max contraction   80% elongation & max contraction

Fig. 3. (Left) FE simulated muscle contractile shape (blue) versus statistical model prediction (red). (Right) FE simulated muscle strain versus statistical model prediction. (Color figure online)

4   Discussion

This study has shown that pre-computing FE simulations of muscle mechanics and capturing this data in a statistical look-up table through Partial Least Squares Regression is an efficient way to automatically predict continuum muscle information. Our PLSR based models predicted shape (within 0.063 mm RMS), force (within 1%), and strain (within 8% max error during contraction). This method rapidly re-creates the 3D muscle with all parameters and accounts for 3D muscle interactions and muscle wrapping around bone and other soft tissues.

While the statistical model predicted musculo-tendon force, muscle shape and muscle strain vector fields accurately, it did not predict the high magnitudes of peak strain in some spatial locations as well. We are currently exploring additional non-linear prediction methods including quadratic PLSR, which may account for some of the non-linear behaviour typically observed in large deformation finite elastic mechanics.

In this study, we used DTI to describe a subject's muscle mechanics but can easily replace this with other imaging modalities including 3D freehand ultrasound. Recent numerical methods that predict fibres based on computational fluid dynamics [15] may also be efficient alternatives. Importantly, the presented framework may play a role in addressing computational cost of predicting detailed muscle information through popular rigid body solvers such as OpenSIM.

References

1. Nielsen, P.M., et al.: Mathematical model of geometry and fibrous structure of the heart. Am. J. Physiol. **260**(4 Pt. 2), H1365–H1378 (1991)
2. Hunter, P.J., et al.: Modeling the mechanical properties of cardiac muscle. Prog. Biophys. Mol. Biol. **69**(2–3), 289–331 (1998)
3. Hunter, P.J., et al.: An anatomical heart model with applications to myocardial activation and ventricular mechanics. Crit. Rev. Biomed. Eng. **20**(5–6), 403–426 (1992)
4. Lemos, R.R., et al.: A framework for structured modeling of skeletal muscle. Comput. Methods Biomech. Biomed. Eng. **7**(6), 305–317 (2004)
5. Agur, A.M., et al.: Documentation and three-dimensional modelling of human soleus muscle architecture. Clin. Anat. **16**(4), 285–293 (2003)
6. Lin, Y.C., et al.: Two-dimensional surrogate contact modeling for computationally efficient dynamic simulation of total knee replacements. J. Biomech. Eng. **131**(4), 041010 (2009)
7. Zhang, J., et al.: Predictive statistical models of baseline variations in 3-D femoral cortex morphology. Med. Eng. Phys. **38**(5), 450–457 (2016)
8. Zhang, J., et al.: Lower limb estimation from sparse landmarks using an articulated shape model. J. Biomech. **49**(16), 3875–3881 (2016)
9. Stejskal, E.O., et al.: Spin diffusion measurements: spin echoes in the presence of time-dependent field gradient. J. Chem. Phys. **42**(1), 288–292 (1965)
10. Fernandez, J.W., et al.: Anatomically based geometric modelling of the musculo-skeletal system and other organs. Biomech. Model. Mechanobiol. **2**(3), 139–155 (2004)
11. Hunter, P., et al.: Integration from proteins to organs: the IUPS Physiome Project. Mech. Ageing Dev. **126**(1), 187–192 (2005)

12. Fernandez, J.W., et al.: An anatomically based patient-specific finite element model of patella articulation: towards a diagnostic tool. Biomech. Model. Mechanobiol. **4**(1), 20–38 (2005)
13. Kim, H.J., et al.: Evaluation of predicted knee-joint muscle forces during gait using an instrumented knee implant. J. Orthop. Res. **27**(10), 1326–1331 (2009)
14. Mateos-Aparicio, G.: Partial Least Squares (PLS) methods: origins, evolution, and application to social sciences. Commun. Stat. Theory Methods **40**(13), 2305–2317 (2011)
15. Handsfield, G.G., et al.: Determining skeletal muscle architecture with Laplacian simulations: a comparison with diffusion tensor imaging. Biomech. Model Mechanobiol. (2 June 2017). doi:10.1007/s10237-017-0923-5

Approaches to Brain Tissue Quantification with Comparison on Supporting the Detection of Age-Related Dementia in MRI

Peifang Guo$^{(\boxtimes)}$

Montreal, QC, Canada
peif.guo@gmail.com

Abstract. In this paper, a comparison of two different approaches is given for brain tissue segmentation using various sources of techniques, the level-set thresholding segmentation with sparse model (LTSSM) and the segmentation with the k-means clustering (SKMC), in magnetic resonance imaging (MRI). In the LTSSM approach, the system searches for level-set thresholding in the working subsets recursively for segmentation. Unlike the LTSSM approach, the SKMC approach applies the k-means clustering to group the brain tissue objects into three classes (grey matter, white matter and cerebrospinal fluid), and then segment the three groups in the different components in the RGB color space. At the validation stage, both approaches of the LTSSM and the SKMC are implemented using the real-time OASIS data for comparison purpose. The experimental results demonstrate the robustness of both approaches for brain tissue segmentation with comparison, in terms of the Dice similarity and sensitivity in MRI.

Keywords: Tissue segmentation · Level-set thresholding · The k-means clustering · Greyscale histogram · Dice similarity · Magnetic resonance imaging

1 Introduction

Medical studies have shown that the degree of atrophy for the volume of brain tissues, e.g., grey matter (GM), could provide an indicator of disease progression for patients with age-related dementia in magnetic resonance imaging (MRI) (Guo 2017; Pepe et al. 2013; Petersen 2003). As the tissue segmentation is a crucial early step in the analysis of brain images, it has become one of the important areas of research in developmental neuroscience (Tohka 2014; Duchesne et al. 2008; Khademi et al. 2012).

One popular category of brain tissue segmentation methods is based on utilizing geometric information such as deformable models using a minimization of an energy functional (West et al. 2012; Yushkevich et al. 2006). A review of some methods can be found in the work (Weiner et al. 2013; Jack et al. 2010; Liew and Hong 2006). Therefore, it may be useful to explore new automatic methods using different sources of techniques for brain tissue segmentation (Masood and Al-Jumaily 2014; Duyn 2012).

The sparsity techniques have been explored for the image shape modeling (Zhang et al. 2012; Hoyer 2004). The goal of the k-means clustering algorithm is to group objects of interest into a known number of categories or *classes* (Demsar 2006). In this

© Springer International Publishing AG 2017
M.J. Cardoso et al. (Eds.): BIVPCS/POCUS 2017, LNCS 10549, pp. 78–85, 2017.
DOI: 10.1007/978-3-319-67552-7_10

study, a comparison of two different approaches is given for brain tissue segmentation using various sources of techniques, the level-set thresholding segmentation with sparsity model (LTSSM) and the segmentation with the k-means clustering (SKMC), in terms of segmentation performance in MRI.

2 Approaches

The histogram based approaches are widely used for image analysis and segmentation, because of the efficiency of the histogram-based techniques (Rafael and Wood 2008; Guo and Bhattacharya 2014). Figure 1 shows the two proposed approaches, the LTSSM and the SKMC, for brain tissue segmentation in MRI for comparison purpose. At the beginning, both of the LTSSM and the SKMC approaches undertake the same operations of image greyscale transformation. The LTSSM approach searches for image thresholds recursively in each of the working subsets to obtain the best resulting segmented brain GM and WM. Unlike the LTSSM approach, the SKMC approach uses the k-means clustering to group classes of white matter (WM), GM and cerebrospinal fluid (CSF) in the RGB (red, green, blue) space, and then segment three clusters of WM, GM and CSF in the three components of R, G and B individually.

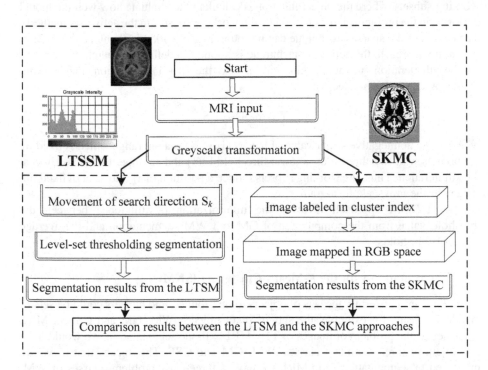

Fig. 1. Approaches of the LTSSM and the SKMC for brain tissue segmentation. (Color figure online)

During the implementation, we validate the methods of the LTSSM and the SKMC on the real-time Open Access Series of Imaging Studies (OASIS) data of brain MRI scans (http://www.oasis-brains.org). In the next subsections, we provide descriptions of both methods of the LTSSM and the SKMC.

2.1 Level-Set Thresholding Segmentation with Sparse Model (LTSSM)

The LTSSM approach is performed alone the search direction, Sk, in the subsets of bin ranges (fixed by thresholds) in the greyscale histogram. Let $r(k)$ be the average value of a lower threshold $Lt(k)$ and an upper threshold $Ut(k)$. At the kth iteration, the $Lt(k)$ and $Ut(k)$ are thus represented by:

$$Lt(k) = r(k+1) - \frac{\{1 - r(k+1)\}}{2}, \text{and}$$
$$Ut(k) = r(k+1) + \frac{\{1 - r(k+1)\}}{2}. \tag{1}$$

We denote the term of x_k as a bin range at the kth iteration, which is fixed by the Lt (k) and $Ut(k)$ in the greyscale histogram.

With the search direction, the process of LTSSM moves recursively on each of the working subsets, where the object function is calculated to evaluate how well the model performs in the problem environment (i.e., the working subsets in the active-set method). The details of the sparsity technique can be found in the work of (Zhang et al. 2012).

In the approach, the active-set technique is applied to define the search direction S_k (at the kth iteration) in the working subsets. At the $(k + 1)$th iteration, the working subset of x_{k+1} is formulated as:

$$x_{k+1} = x_k + \alpha \times S_k, \tag{2}$$

where α is a nonnegative scalar value of bin. x_k ($x_k \in \mathbf{X}$) is a bin range which is fixed by the bounds with two thresholds, a lower threshold $Lt(k)$ and an upper threshold $Ut(k)$ at the kth iteration. Thus, the working subsets induce a partition of x_k into a set of fixed bin ranges in the greyscale histogram.

The LTSSM approach involves the minimization of difference between the threshold value from the computation of GM and WM segmentation and the average value of thresholds.

2.2 Segmentation with the K-Means Clustering (SKMC)

In the k-means clustering, the sets of objects to be grouped into clusters could be sets of physical objects, for example, the sets of pixel objects, WM, GM and CSF in MRI. Considering the problem of images of T1w MRI in tissue segmentation, we would have a problem of three dominant classes, WM, GM and CSF. This means that if we are interested in segmentation from MRI, we have a three-class problem (classes of WM, GM and CSF) during the k-means clustering with $k = 3$.

In the SKMC approach, we assume that the data of brain images are estimated approximately with three dominant classes, corresponding to the WM, GM and CSF.

During the k-means clustering, we label each of image pixel objects in MRI into three clusters (WM, GM and CSF) in greyscale; since the greyscale is the summation of vectors of R, G and B, we further map the labeled images into the RGB color space.

3 Implementation

During the implementation, we validate the two approaches, the LTSSM and the SKMC, on the real-time OASIS data of brain MRI scans. On the OASIS data, each subject has three to four T1w images, averaged in order to improve the signal/noise ratio. All 198 MRI subjects on the OASIS data are right-handed, where images were aligned within the Talairach reference frame via affine transform T.

3.1 The LTSSM Segmentation Results

Figure 2 shows an example of the experiments on the OASIS in the LTSSM implementation. Figure 2(a) is the raw images, and Fig. 2(b) is the greyscale histograms, showing three dominant modes corresponding to the two types of tissues (from the right: WM and GM), and CSF.

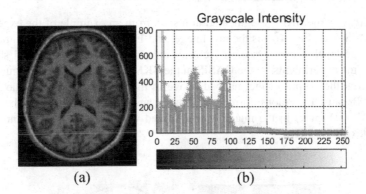

(a)   (b)

Fig. 2. An example of the experiments on the OASIS in the LTSSM implementation; from the left row: (a) raw images; (b) image greyscale histograms.

In the LTSSM evaluation process, we compute the $Lt(k)$ and $Ut(k)$, (see Eq. (1)) recursively in each likelihood threshold-based region x_k ($x_k \in X$), fixed by $[Lt(k), Ut(k)]$, in the histograms. The S_k (see Eq. (2)) is equal to '+1' because the propagation direction is defined from the left to the right in the one-dimensional histograms. We select the nonnegative scalar α (see Eq. (3)) in a bin-width of 5, rather than of 1, in order to avoid unnecessary computation of $D(k)$ (see Eq. (3)) in the evaluation. The results of the evaluation process are the two 2-D arrays of $D(k)\{Lt(k), Ut(k)\}$, corresponding the two types of GM and WM tissues.

Finally, the application of the LTSSM procedure in segmentation resulted in the optimal bin ranges of [30, 70] for the GM and [70, 100] for the WM on the OASIS.

Figure 3 presents the LTSSM implementation results from an example of the experiments on the OASIS in their optimal bin range solutions for tissue segmentation of the GM (see Fig. 3(a)) and the WM (see Fig. 3(b)), each with color lines in the left and grey color in the right.

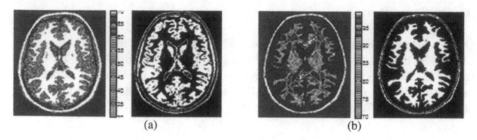

(a)   (b)

Fig. 3. An example of the experiments on the OASIS in the LTSSM implementation: (a) the GM segmentation results in the optimal bin range [30, 70], and (b) the WM segmentation results in the optimal bin range [70, 100], with the color lines in the left and the grey color in the right. (Color figure online)

3.2   The SKMC Segmentation Results

Figure 4 presents the SKMC segmentation results from an example of the experiments on the OASIS data; Fig. 4(a) is the raw image, and Fig. 4(b) displays the output of the sample image labeled in greyscale by cluster index in clustering. Figure 5 shows an example of the experiments on the OASIS in the SKMC implementation. Figure 5(a) is obtained from the output of the mapped image in the RGB space during the k-means clustering. Because the color information of the image in Fig. 5(a) exists in the space of 'R' 'G' 'B', each pixel in the image is categorized with a value of R, G and B in its cluster index in the MRI.

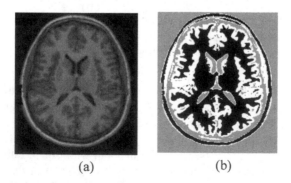

(a)   (b)

Fig. 4. An example of the experiments on the real-time OASIS data in the SKMC implementation; (a) the raw image; (b) output of the labeled image by cluster index during the clustering.

By using the Euclidean distance to measure how close pixel objects are to each other, the *k*-means clustering involved in the ISKC-PS approach then returns an index of the color component ('R', or 'G', or 'B'), corresponding to a cluster (WM, or GM, or CSF) in the image; Fig. 5(b) presents the implementation results from an example of the experiments on the OASIS, where the clusters of WM, GM and CSF (from the left to the right) in the RGB color space are segmented individually in the 'R', 'G' and 'B' components.

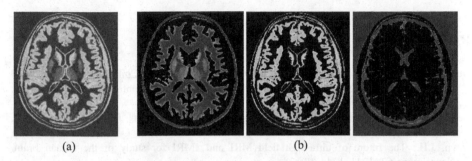

(a)   (b)

Fig. 5. An example of the experiments on the OASIS in the SKMC implementation; (a) output of the mapped image in the RGB space during clustering; (b) results of segmented WM, GM and CSF (from the left to the right) in the components of 'R', 'G' and 'B' individually.

3.3   Comparison Results

In the comparison, the Dice similarity (DI) index are utilized in order to assess the capability of different methods qualitatively for tissue segmentation in brain MRI:

$$DI = \frac{2 \times TP}{2 \times TP + FP + FN} \times 100\%, \tag{3}$$

where TP, FP and FN denote true positive (or sensitivity), false positive and false negative, respective.

In terms of the DI, TP and true negative (TN, or specificity), Table 1 shows the comparison results between the proposed approaches of the LTSSM and the SKMC on the OASIS data. As shown in Table 1, the performance for both of the LTSSM and SKMC approaches for classification of GM and WM are about on a par in terms of TN, where the SKMC obtained the higher rate of 83.83% for WM while the LTSSM obtained the lower rate of 82.45% for WM in segmentation. It also can be observe that, from Table 1, the difference of DI among the methods for the segmented GM and WM is ranged from 80.34% to 83.25%. In addition, overall, the proposed SKMC approach achieves higher rates of DI and TP in segmentation performance, compared with those obtained by the LTSSM approach.

Table 1. Comparison results between the proposed approaches of the LTSSM and the SKMC

Methods	WM/GM (DI %)	WM/GM (TP %)	WM/GM (TN %)
LTSSM	80.75/80.34	81.98/80.92	82.45/83.76
SKMC	81.25/81.05	82.32/81.76	83.83/83.81

4 Conclusion

In this study, the experimental results demonstrate the robustness of both approaches of the LTSSM and the SKMC with different techniques for brain tissue segmentation in MRI. Our future work will also be dedicated to examining the robustness of approaches of both LTSSM and SKMC to large data of MRI samples for quantitative analysis in the volumes of brain tissues clinically.

References

Duchesne, S., Caroli, A., Geroldi, C., Barillot, C., Frisoni, G.B., Collins, D.L.: MRI based automated computer classification of probable ad versus normal controls. IEEE Trans. Med. Imaging **27**, 509–520 (2008)

Demsar, J.: Statistical comparisons of classifiers over multiple data sets. J. Mach. Learn. Res. **7**, 1–30 (2006)

Duyn, J.H.: The future of ultra-high field MRI and fMRI for study of the human brain. Neuroimage **62**, 1241–1248 (2012)

Guo, P.: A tissue-based biomarker model for predicting disease patterns. J. Knowl. Based Syst. **276**, 160–169 (2017)

Guo, P., Bhattacharya, P.: An evolutionary framework for detecting protein conformation defects. J. Inf. Sci. **276**, 332–342 (2014)

Hoyer, P.O.: Non-negative matrix factorization with sparseness constraints. J. Mach. Learn. Res. **5**, 1457–1469 (2004)

Jack Jr., C.R., Knopman, D.S., Jagust, W.J., Shaw, L.M., Aisen, P.S., Weiner, M.W., Petersen, R.C., Trojanowski, J.Q.: Hypothetical model of dynamic biomarkers of the Alzheimer's pathological cascade. Lancet Neurol. **9**, 119–128 (2010)

Khademi, A., Venetsanopoulos, A., Moody, A.R.: Robust white matter lesion segmentation in FLAIR MRI. IEEE Trans. Biomed. Eng. **2012**(59), 860–871 (2012)

Liew, A.W.C., Hong, Y.: Current methods in automatic tissue segmentation of 3D magnetic resonance brain images. Current Med. Imaging Rev. **2**(1), 91–103 (2006)

Masood, A., Al-Jumaily, A.A.: Computer aided diagnostic support system for skin cancer: a review of techniques and algorithms. J. Biomed. Engineering **2013**, 122–132 (2014)

Pepe, A., Zhao, L., Koikkalainen, J., Hietala, J., Ruotsalainen, U., Tohka, J.: Automatic statistical shape analysis of cerebral asymmetry in 3D T1-weighted magnetic resonance images at vertex-level: application to neuroleptic-naïve schizophrenia. Magn. Reson. Imaging **31**, 676–687 (2013)

Petersen, R.C.: Mild Cognitive Impairment: Aging to Alzheimer's Disease. Oxford University Press, New York (2003)

Rafael, R.C., Wood, R.E.: Digital Image Processing, 3rd edn. Prentice Hall, Upper Saddle River (2008)

Tohka, J.: Partial volume effect modeling for segmentation and tissue classification of brain magnetic resonance images: a review. World J. Radiol. **11**, 855–864 (2014)

West, J., Warntjes, J.B., Lundberg, P.: Novel whole brain segmentation and volume estimation using quantitative MRI. Eur. Radiol. **2012**(22), 998–1007 (2012)

Weiner, M.W., Veitch, D.P., Aisen, P.S., Beckett, L.A., Cairns, N.J., Green, R.C., Harvey, D., Jack, C.R., Jagust, W., Liu, E., Morris, J.C., Petersen, R.C., Saykin, A.J., Schmidt, M.E., Shaw, L., Shen, L., Siuciak, J.A., Soares, H., Toga, A.W., Trojanowski, J.Q.: The Alzheimer's disease neuroimaging initiative: a review of papers published since its inception. Alzheimers Dement **9**, e111–e194 (2013)

Yushkevich, P.A., Piven, J., Hazlett, H.C., Smith, R.G., Ho, S., Gee, J.C., Gerig, G.: User-guided 3D active contour segmentation of anatomical structures: significantly improved efficiency and reliability. NeuroImage **31**, 1116–1128 (2006)

Zhang, S., Zhan, Y., Dewan, M., Huang, J., Metaxas, D.N., Zhou, X.S.: Towards robust and effective shape modeling: sparse shape composition. Med. Image Anal. **16**, 265–277 (2012)

Relating Atrial Appendage Flow Stasis Risk from Computational Fluid Dynamics to Imaging Based Appearance Paradigms for Cardioembolic Risk

Soroosh Sanatkhani[1] and Prahlad G. Menon[1,2]([X])

[1] Department of Bioengineering, University of Pittsburgh,
Pittsburgh, PA 15219, USA
[2] Department of Biomedical Engineering, Duquesne University,
Pittsburgh, PA 15282, USA
menongopalakrip@duq.edu

Abstract. Emboli originating from the left atrial appendage are a major cause of transient ischemic attack and cardioembolic stroke. Whereas this risk has been shown to be correlated with left atrial appendage morphology (Cactus, Chicken Wing, Windsock, and Cauliflower shapes) determined from 3D imaging, this clinical correlation is found wanting with regard to a biomechanically grounded underlying basis for thrombosis based on intra-atrial hemodynamics. We define a novel probabilistic risk stratification paradigm for intra-atrial flow stasis based on personalized computational fluid dynamics.

Keywords: Computational fluid dynamics · Flow stasis · Cardioembolic risk · Left atrial appendage morphology

1 Introduction

In the presence of atrial fibrillation (AF), reduced cardiac contractility results in flow stasis and thrombus formation, which in-turn increases the risk of cardioembolic complications and stroke. The left atrial appendage (LAA) is hypothesized to be the principal location for intra-atrial thrombus formation [1, 2] in approximately 2.3 million US adults with AF [3], putting them at risk of cardioembolic stroke [2, 4, 5]. This provides clinical rationale for exclusion/occlusion of the LAA in the interest of reducing the risk of stroke. Currently most stroke and thromboembolism (TE) risk predictions for AF patients are based on clinical risk stratification schemes like Framingham, NICE, ChadS$_2$ and CHA$_2$DS$_2$-VASc which are developed by series of risk factors identified from trial cohorts [6]. Even more refined versions of these schemes [7] do not determine stroke risk of an individual based on the patient-specific hemodynamics and physics. In an attempt to stratify patient-specific stroke risk, the LAA appearance has been classified into four unique categories (viz. Chicken-Wing, Windsock, Cactus and Cauliflower appearance) to assist with preoperative planning for LAA occlusion/exclusion based on some geometrical features such as existence of obvious bend, LAA length, number of lobes and etc. [8] and correlated with stroke risk

© Springer International Publishing AG 2017
M.J. Cardoso et al. (Eds.): BIVPCS/POCUS 2017, LNCS 10549, pp. 86–93, 2017.
DOI: 10.1007/978-3-319-67552-7_11

by considering clinical mortality statistics [9]. However, the relation between the LAA morphology and stroke risk is not well defined and some studies have reported this classification as being non-longitudinal for stasis stratification [10]. Further, while the effect of atrial geometry on AF has received some attention in the literature [11], the influence of patient-specific LAA shape on hemodynamics of stasis has not been quantitatively analyzed. A hemodynamic model of the LA can help objectify decisions making regarding the existence of regional stasis (and therefore cardioembolic stroke) risk, which in-turn may help with oral anticoagulant (OAC) management for patients with low CHA_2DS_2-VaSc and help guide therapeutic choices of intervention [9]. To develop such a stasis risk stratification tool, we employ computational fluid dynamics (CFD) to model probability of red blood cell (RBC) residence in the LAA and study LAA-specific residence time distributions (RTD) for 8 AF patients. The remainder of this paper is organized as follows: we present our methodology to segment LA geometries from patient-specific medical images to surface geometries, followed by our CFD modeling approach for transient particle transport and stasis probability computation from RTD data, and finally present results & conclusions from a comparative analysis of unique patient-specific LAA geometries in our cohort, using our RTD-based stasis probability scores.

2 Methods

2.1 Image Segmentation

Contrast-enhanced cardiac computed tomography (CCT) DICOM images of 8 AF patients having unique LAA morphologies, were iteratively segmented in 3D to extract the LA surface, including LAA and pulmonary venous inlets (including up to 2 inlet diameters), until the mitral valve plane (excluding valvular structures), using a basic iso-contouring approach, in Paraview (Kitware Inc.), followed by surface preparation steps, including regional smoothing and definition of flat inlets and outlet planes in Geomagic Studio 10 (Geomagic Inc.), in order to result in surface models suitable for computational flow studies.

2.2 Mesh Preparation

To determine the maximum mesh element size, we calculated the Taylor micro-scale (λ) which is in between the largest and smallest length vortical scales. The mitral valve outlet diameter ranged from 1.9–3.1 cm, making the minimum turbulence length scale, $l = 0.07D = 1.33$ mm. The assumed overall venous inflow rate of 2 L/min makes $U_{max} = \frac{2Q}{A} = 0.235$ m/s and the turbulent kinetic energy, $k = \frac{3}{2}(UI)^2 = 3.547 \times 10^{-4} \frac{J}{kg}$, where I is a function of Reynolds number. Using the $k - \varepsilon$ model, the energy dissipation rate is assumed $\varepsilon = (0.09)^{\frac{3}{4}} k^{\frac{3}{2}} l^{-1} = 8.254 \times 10^{-4} \frac{J}{kg.s}$ [12]. Therefore, the Taylor micro-scale will be, $\lambda = \sqrt{10\nu \frac{k}{\varepsilon}} = 3.878$ mm. So, the maximum element size in our mesh was set to 3.5 mm. Further, to establish grid-independence for CFD studies, we calculated the energy dissipation rate of the atrium and increased the mesh density until changes were less than 5%. The final blood-contacting volume were meshed in 3D with ~250000–450000 tetrahedral elements including layered boundary fitted inflation grids with prismatic elements, generated using the meshing utilities in ANSYS Workbench 18 (Fig. 1).

2.3   Global CFD Assumptions

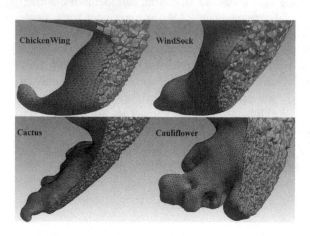

Fig. 1. Unique LAA morphologies from the study cohort showing 3D tetrahedral mesh elements.

Two separate series of simulations were conducted in this study. The first was with a cohort of 4 AF patients, employing a coupled version of unsteady flow and unsteady scalar transport, implemented using a modified solved in OpenFOAM. The second was with a larger cohort of 8 AF patients using pre-solved steady flow field as an input to unsteady scalar transport solver. Incompressible Newtonian blood flow with rigid, impermeable walls (simulative of idealized AF conditions) ($\mu = 0.00371$ Pa.s, $\rho = 1060$ kg/m^3) was assumed throughout both simulation series'. Further, the mitral valve was considered to be open during all simulations.

2.4   Unsteady Flow Model

Probability of stasis was quantified by examining the RTD obtained by modeling purely convective transport of a pulse of neutrally buoyant particles (viz. RBCs) injected at the pulmonary inlet, after ~35 cardiac cycles. An unsteady flow scalar transport solver (developed from IcoFoam and ScalarTransportFoam, in OpenFOAM), employed for simulation. LAA-specific RTD are established by using mean instantaneous particle density in the LAA as a proxy for the probability of a particle being present in the LAA after a given period of time. To calculate the RTD, we injected a Kronecker delta function of scalar concentration of unity (representative of RBCs) at each of the four pulmonary venous inlets, with an injection pulse width of 0.01 s at the beginning of the pulsatile pulmonary venous flow shifted waveform [13] (Fig. 2). The waveform was delayed in a manner such that atrial systole took place at the end of each cycle. Diffusion coefficient for the particles was considered 0 m^2/s (i.e. advection only transport). The time step, dt = 0.25 ms, was considered after a time-step independence study evaluating the solution for time distribution of LAA particle concentration in the WindSock geometry.

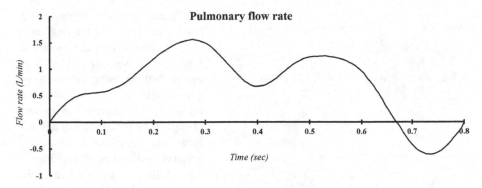

Fig. 2. Pulmonary venous flow waveform utilized at each pulmonary inlet to the LA (from Smiseth et al. [13]).

2.5 Steady Flow Model

Unsteady simulations consume higher computational cost and further since the particles linger for a long time in the LAA relative to the rest of the LAA, observation for up to 35–40 cardiac cycles is required prior to particles movement achieving a stable final state; which adds up to long simulation times per geometry. Therefore, for a larger cohort of 8 AF patients, we attempted to solve for a steady velocity field to initialize an unsteady scalar transport solver in an uncoupled manner, to determine LAA-specific RTDs similar to the previous section.

3 Results and Discussion

The CFD simulation based particle residence were validated against experimental particle image velocimetry results in the WindSock LA geometry (Fig. 3) [14].

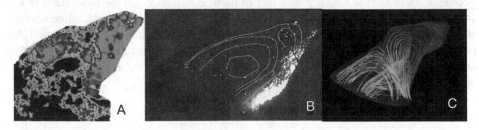

Fig. 3. (A) PIV vector computation result colored with flow velocity magnitude, normalized from minimum (purple for stasis i.e. $|V| = 0$ m/s) to maximum (red), for particles seen in a projection of the illuminated LAA volume. (B) Approximate path-lines of the particles (manually traced as white lines) in the appendage, superimposed on an instantaneous screenshot of the same projection plane. The fluorescent particles in the regions of stasis can be clearly seen, corresponding with purple regions of stasis in the distal LAA regions. (C) CFD generated streamlines of flow in the LAA, colored by velocity magnitude, normalized minimum to maximum (blue to red) [14]. (Color figure online)

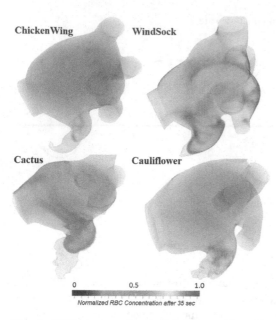

ChickenWing   WindSock

Cactus   Cauliflower

0   0.5   1.0
Normalized RBC Concentration after 35 sec

Fig. 4. RBC concentration in LA after ~ 44 cardiac cycles (i.e. 35 s) indicates highest RBC concentration in the LAA with markedly higher RBC density in the Cauliflower geometry relative to the Chicken Wing LAA.

Spatial particle density (i.e. concentration) distributions after ~ 44 cardiac cycles are plotted in Fig. 4. LAA-specific RTDs were established by using mean instantaneous particle density in the LAA region (i.e. ostium to distal tip) as a proxy for the probability of a RBCs being present in the LAA after a given period of time, evaluating the same 8 times every cardiac cycle, for ~ 44 cycles (35 s).

Comparing RTDs for the modeled LAAs (see Fig. 5) revealed that RBCs enter the LAA relatively more easily and leave more quickly in the Chicken Wing geometry, as evidenced by the lower peak/median RT. RBCs may be relatively more prone to form thrombus inside Cauliflower and Windsock LAAs owing to its relatively higher peak RT and right-skewed RTD. Further, for purposes of comparison, the cohort-averaged RTD for a control volume in the middle of the atrium reveals that LAA of any shape category is more likely to thrombus formation than other regions of atrium, as evidenced by its lower RTD peak/median value.

Table 1 reports the RTD tail-area for RT > 20 s (i.e. 25 cycles), which describes the probability of RBCs being resident in the LAA after 25 cycles. The Chicken Wing geometry again had the lowest probability of particle residence and therefore stasis risk, which is congruent with the clinical literature on LAA appearance-based cardioembolic risk statistics. The common finding among prior clinical studies looking into LA hemodynamics is that Chicken-Wing shaped LAA has the lowest risk of TE [9, 15, 16] so those patients with CHA_2DS_2-VASc < 2 can avoid oral anticoagulant (OAC) therapy for bleeding risk [15].

Table 1. Probability of RBCs remaining in the LAA beyond 25 cardiac cycles, based on CFD for ~ 44 cycles of unsteady and coupled particle transport of a pulse of RBCs injected at the pulmonary venous inlets at the start of atrial diastole.

RTD tail-area (Stasis Probability)	Chicken-Wing	WindSock	Cactus	Cauliflower
LAA Region	0.178	0.186	0.1801	0.203
Control Volume in center of LA	0.017	0.008	0.0002	0.0008

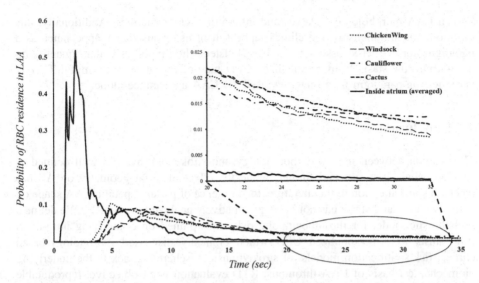

Fig. 5. Superimposed RTD probability density estimates for particles in the LAA volume (i.e. LAA orifice to distal tip) of each unique geometry in our study cohort along with the cohort-averaged RTD for a small central control volume inside LA (solid line), presented 35 s after synchronized injection of the RBC pulses at the pulmonary venous inlets. In each case, the LAA had a higher median residence time (RT) relative to the central intra-atrial control volume.

RTD results with our larger study cohort using the uncoupled RBC transport simulated on an initialized steady CFD velocity field depicted that there is a significant variation in stasis (and therefore, TE risk) between LAAs in a same group (see Fig. 6), which warrants a larger clinical cohort to validate the relationship between the four

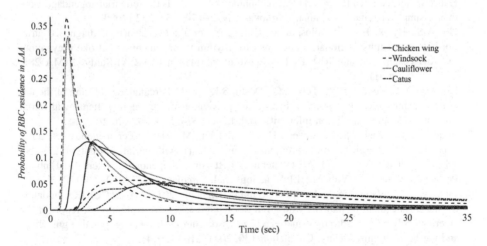

Fig. 6. RTD probability density estimates for RBC concentration in the LAA volume of each unique geometry in our study cohort of 8 AF patients (2 per each group) showing a significant variation in stasis risk prediction (i.e. RTD curves) between LAAs of same group especially for the Windsock and Cauliflower morphologies.

known LAA morphological classes and intra-atrial hemodynamics. Additionally, this questions the simplicity of the clinical approach of using just LAA appearance as a paradigm for TE risk assessment. This bolsters the hypothesis that quantifying intra-atrial flow stasis from personalized CFD may offer a more meaningful TE risk classification paradigm than imaging based 3D LAA appearance alone.

4 Conclusion

The relation between the LAA morphology and stroke risk has not well defined in previous clinical studies and further, while the effect of atrial geometry on AF has received some attention in the literature, the influence of patient-specific LAA shape on hemodynamics and stasis has not been quantitatively analyzed previously. We define a probabilistic model for thromboembolic risk, underpinned on quantifying intra-atrial flow stasis from personalized CFD which clinically discussed morphology-based clinical risk stratification models for stroke/transient ischemic attack to the underlying biomechanical basis of LAA thrombus. RTD evaluation is an objective, reproducible measure to stratify AF patients with regards to stroke risk which directly represents the thrombus risk in a region. This method can improve the patient selection decision for LAA exclusion/occlusion and increase the preciseness of anticoagulant management based on not just shape alone.

References

1. Blackshear, J.L., Odell, J.A.: Appendage obliteration to reduce stroke in cardiac surgical patients with atrial fibrillation. Ann. Thorac. Surg. **61**, 755–759 (1996)
2. Hara, H., Virmani, R., Holmes, D.R., Buchbinder, M., et al.: Is the left atrial appendage more than a simple appendage? Cathet. Cardiovasc. Interv. **74**, 234–242 (2009)
3. Go, A.S., Hylek, E.M., Phillips, K.A., Chang, Y., et al.: Prevalence of diagnosed atrial fibrillation in adults: national implications for rhythm management and stroke prevention: the AnTicoagulation and Risk Factors in Atrial Fibrillation (ATRIA) Study. JAMA **285**, 2370–2375 (2001)
4. Holmes, D.R., Reddy, V.Y., Turi, Z.G., Doshi, S.K., et al.: Percutaneous closure of the left atrial appendage versus warfarin therapy for prevention of stroke in patients with atrial fibrillation: a randomised non-inferiority trial. Lancet **374**, 534–542 (2009)
5. Reddy, V.Y., Doshi, S.K., Sievert, H., Buchbinder, M., et al.: Percutaneous left atrial appendage closure for stroke prophylaxis in patients with atrial fibrillation 2.3-year follow-up of the PROTECT AF (Watchman Left Atrial Appendage System for Embolic Protection in Patients With Atrial Fibrillation) trial. Circulation **127**, 720–729 (2013)
6. January, C.T., Wann, L.S., Alpert, J.S., Calkins, H., et al.: 2014 AHA/ACC/HRS guideline for the management of patients with atrial fibrillation: executive summary. A report of the american college of cardiology/american heart association task force on practice guidelines and the heart rhythm society. Circulation **130**, 2071–2104 (2014)
7. Lip, G.Y.H., Nieuwlaat, R., Pisters, R., Lane, D.A., et al.: Refining clinical risk stratification for predicting stroke and thromboembolism in atrial fibrillation using a novel risk factor-based approach: the euro heart survey on atrial fibrillation. Chest **137**, 263–272 (2010)

8. Wang, Y.A.N., Di Biase, L., Horton, R.P., Nguyen, T., et al.: Left atrial appendage studied by computed tomography to help planning for appendage closure device placement. J. Cardiovasc. Electrophysiol. **21**, 973–982 (2010)
9. Di Biase, L., Santangeli, P., Anselmino, M., Mohanty, P., et al.: Does the left atrial appendage morphology correlate with the risk of stroke in patients with atrial fibrillation?: Results from a multicenter study. J. Am. Coll. Cardiol. **60**, 531–538 (2012)
10. Khurram, I.M., Dewire, J., Mager, M., Maqbool, F., et al.: Relationship between left atrial appendage morphology and stroke in patients with atrial fibrillation. Heart Rhythm **10**, 1843–1849 (2013)
11. Krueger, M.W., Rhode, K.S., O'Neill, M.D., Rinaldi, C.A., et al.: Patient-specific modeling of atrial fibrosis increases the accuracy of sinus rhythm simulations and may explain maintenance of atrial fibrillation. J. Electrocardiol. **47**, 324–328 (2014)
12. Kim, S.-W., Chen, Y.-S.: Computation of turbulent boundary layer flows with an algebraic stress turbulence model (1986)
13. Smiseth, O.A., Thompson, C.R., Lohavanichbutr, K., Ling, H., et al.: The pulmonary venous systolic flow pulse—its origin and relationship to left atrial pressure. J. Am. Coll. Cardiol. **34**, 802–809 (1999)
14. Sanatkhani, S., Finoli, M., Shroff, S.G., Menon, P.G.: Visualization of patient-specific hemodynamics in atrial fibrillation using computational and experimental models. In: Xie, X., Nithiarasu, P., Robertson, A., Etienne, B., Sazonov, I., Xie, X. (eds.) 5th International Conference on Computational & Mathematical Biomedical Engineering, pp. 432–435. CMBE (2017)
15. Lupercio, F., Diaz, J.C., Spinetto, P.V., Briceno, D., et al.: Left atrial appendage morphology and stroke risk in patients with atrial fibrillation: a meta-analysis. J. Am. Coll. Cardiol. **67**, 713 (2016)
16. Fukushima, K., Fukushima, N., Kato, K., Ejima, K., et al.: Correlation between left atrial appendage morphology and flow velocity in patients with paroxysmal atrial fibrillation. Eur. Heart J. Cardiovasc. Imaging **17**, 59–66 (2016)

Deformable Multi-material 2-Simplex Surface Mesh for Intraoperative MRI-Ready Surgery Planning and Simulation, with Deep-Brain Stimulation Applications

T. Rashid[1], S. Sultana[1], G.S. Fischer[2], J. Pilitsis[3], and M.A. Audette[1(✉)]

[1] Old Dominion University, Norfolk, USA
maudette@odu.edu
[2] Worcester Polytechnic Institute, Worcester, USA
[3] Albany Medical Center, Albany, USA

Abstract. Printed and/or digital atlases are important tools for medical research and surgical intervention. While these atlases can provide guidance in identifying anatomical structures, they do not take into account the wide variations in the shape and size of anatomical structures that can occur from patient to patient. Accurate, patient-specific representations are especially important for surgical interventions like deep brain stimulation, where even small inaccuracies can result in dangerous complications. This research effort extends the discrete deformable 2-simplex mesh into the multi-material domain where geometry-based internal forces and image-based external forces are used in the deformation process. Multi-material 2-simplex meshes having shared boundaries are initialized from multi-material triangular surface meshes. A multi-material deformable framework is presented and used to segment anatomical structures of the deep brain region such as the subthalamic nucleus.

Keywords: Segmentation · 2-Simplex mesh · Multi-material · Basal ganglia

1 Introduction

Printed and digital atlases are important tools for medical interventions. While these atlases can provide reasonable guidance in identifying anatomical structures, they do not take into account the large variations in the shape and size of anatomical structures that occur from patient to patient. An accurate depiction of the anatomy is especially important for surgical interventions like deep brain stimulation, where even small inaccuracies can result in potentially dangerous complications. In these situations, a patient-specific representation of the anatomical structures of interest is preferred, rather than a generic printed or digital atlas. Deformable surface meshes are one way to achieve such patient-specific representations. An initial mesh model of the structures of interest can be generated using a digital atlas, and then deformed using patient-specific CT or MR data. Not only is the deformed multi-surface mesh capable of accurately representing the structures of interest, this mesh is sparser than volumetric representations, such as tetrahedral or hexahedral meshes, and thus reduces computational overhead. This work

M.J. Cardoso et al. (Eds.): BIVPCS/POCUS 2017, LNCS 10549, pp. 94–102, 2017.
DOI: 10.1007/978-3-319-67552-7_12

presents an extension of the discrete deformable 2-simplex mesh. The innovation here is a multi-material implementation of deformable meshes which can be initialized with relative ease and deformed using MRI data to accurately segment anatomical structures of the deep brain region, while imposing continuous motion through various functional structures. This applies to both introperative MRI-ready surgery planning and anatomical modeling with shared surfaces for surgery simulation.

1.1 Background and Motivation

Delingette formulated a specific type of deformable model: the k-simplex mesh [1] for 3D shape reconstruction and segmentation. A k-simplex mesh is defined as a k-manifold discrete mesh where each vertex is linked to exactly $k + 1$ neighboring vertices. Delingette specifies a *simplex angle* and *metric parameters*, which can be used to represent the position of any vertex with respect to its neighbors. 2-Simplex meshes are dual to triangular meshes. Simplex forces, comprised of *internal* forces are based on mesh geometry and *external* forces are based on input image gradients, together with enhancements such as shape constraints, smoothing parameters, shape memory constraints [2] and statistical shape information [3] have allowed simplex meshes to be used for accurate segmentation of anatomical structures. Gilles introduced a multi-surface 2-simplex model with collision detection and handling to segment muscles and bone from MRI data [2]. In the above, the 2-simplex surface meshes were used to represent singular structures.

In this paper, we extend the 2-simplex model to achieve multi-material deformable meshes consisting of two or more *sub-meshes*, where each sub-mesh bounds a specific structure. The shared boundary between sub-meshes is consistent and removes any possibility of volume overlap between sub-meshes. Our contribution is a method to produce a deformable multi-surface mesh atlas from a voxel-based 3D digital atlas.

2 Methods

A 2-simplex model is 2-manifold discrete mesh where every vertex is connected to three neighboring vertices. It undergoes deformations based on geometry-based internal forces and image-based external forces, using the Newtonian law of motion [1]:

$$m_i \frac{d^2 P_i}{dt^2} = -\gamma \frac{dP_i}{dt} + F_{int} + F_{ext} \tag{1}$$

where m_i is the mass, and P_i is the position of a vertex of the mesh. F_{int} represents all internal forces and F_{ext} represents all the image-based, gradient-attracted external forces acting on P_i, while γ represents a damping coefficient.

2.1   Initializing a Multi-material 2-Simplex Mesh

A 2-simplex mesh is the topological dual of a triangular mesh [1]. This geometric duality can be exploited to generate 2-simplex meshes from triangular surface meshes. Figure 1 shows an illustration of the duality. The centroids of triangles in the triangular mesh coincide with the vertices of the simplex mesh, and edges of the simplex mesh are created by linking these simplex vertices. In Fig. 1 the red dots on the triangular mesh represents the centroids that eventually become vertices of the 2-simplex mesh. Two assumptions are made when converting a triangular mesh into a simplex mesh:

1. The triangular mesh is assumed to be watertight (no holes or gaps),
2. The triangular mesh is assumed to be 2-manifold.

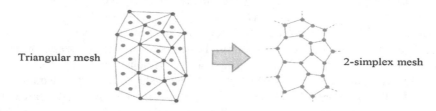

Fig. 1.   Converting a triangular mesh into a simplex mesh (Color figure online)

A closed 2-simplex mesh is a watertight 2-manifold mesh with no gaps and/or boundary edges. On the other hand, a multi-material 2-simplex (MM2S) mesh will contain non-manifold edges and/or vertices. This situation is analogous to the multi-material triangular surface meshes discussed in the previous section. We use a modified version of the Dual Contouring algorithm (DC) [4] to generate multi-material triangular surface meshes, and use these to initialize MM2S meshes.

While the duality between 2-simplex meshes and triangular meshes remains true even for multi-material meshes, the above algorithm needs to be adjusted slightly to account for the multi-material nature of the meshes. The multi-material triangular meshes contain material information associated with triangles, and this information can be exploited to produce MM2S meshes in the following manner:

- Step 1: Compute the centroids of each triangle of the triangular mesh.
- Step 2: For each material index
- Step 2.1: For each ith vertex of the triangular mesh,
  - Step 2.1.1: Locate all triangles with current material index containing i^{th} vertex
  - Step 2.1.2: Use the centroids of these triangles to create one simplex cell.

Since simplex vertices and cells are being created for each material index, care must be taken to avoid duplicate and overlapping cells along the shared boundaries. Figure 2 illustrates the conversion process for a multi-material triangular mesh. Figure 2(a) shows a synthetic box comprising two materials, Fig. 2(b) shows a wireframe rendering of the box. The red colored part of the mesh represents one material while the blue colored part represents the second. The green colored part of the mesh represents the shared boundary. Figure 2(c) and (d) show the multi-material 2-simplex and its wireframe.

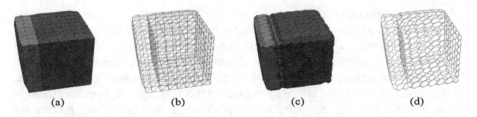

(a)	(b)	(c)	(d)

Fig. 2. Converting a multi-material triangular mesh into a multi-material 2-simplex mesh. (Color figure online)

2.2 Description of Multi-material 2-Simplex Meshes

The multi-material nature of the triangular surface meshes were described by assigning pairwise material indices to triangles. Since the vertices of 2-simplex meshes are dual to triangles in triangular meshes, it is reasonable to assign the triangles' pairwise material indices to their corresponding dual vertices in the 2-simplex mesh. This procedure ensures the preservation of material information in the conversion process. The number of vertices of the 2-simplex mesh will be the same as the number of triangles in the triangular mesh. Furthermore, a MM2S mesh will have shared boundaries as well as non-manifold edges and vertices. Because of its multi-material nature, this type of a k-simplex mesh is not a true 2-simplex mesh in the sense that vertices along the non-manifold edges of the shared boundary can have more than 3 neighboring vertices.

A MM2S mesh can be described as the set $\mathbf{S}^M$ where $\mathbf{V}$ is the set of n vertices with $\mathbf{M}$ being the set of positive integers describing material indices, and p and q are the pairwise material indices assigned to each vertex. $\mathbf{E}$ is the set of m edges.

$$\mathbf{S}^M = \{\mathbf{V}, \mathbf{E}\} \tag{2}$$

$$\begin{aligned} &\{v_i^{p,q}\}, \{i = 0, \dots, n\}, v_i \in \mathbb{R}^3, \{p, q \in \mathbf{M}\}, p \neq q, \mathbf{M} \in \mathbb{N}^+ \\ &\{\{v_i, v_j\}_m\}, \forall v_i \in \mathbf{V}, \forall v_j \in \mathbf{V}, i \neq j \end{aligned} \tag{3}$$

Each material sub-mesh of a multi-material simplex mesh is a pure 2-simplex mesh in the sense that all vertices of the sub-mesh have exactly 3 neighboring vertices. This aspect of the MM2S mesh can be exploited when performing deformation of the mesh.

2.3 Overview of Deformable Multi-material 2-Simplex Meshes

Once the initial MM2S mesh is generated from the triangular mesh, it is split into its constituent sub-meshes. Both the MM2S mesh and its sub-meshes are kept in memory. As mentioned above, each sub-mesh is a pure 2-simplex mesh where every vertex is connected to exactly three neighboring vertices. For every iteration of deformation, internal and external forces are computed. Internal forces are based on mesh geometry, and external forces are based on an input image or volume. The forces are then used to separately deform each sub-mesh sequentially using the mesh evolution process [2].

Since forces are computed independently of sub-meshes, the corresponding vertices making up the shared boundary may not necessarily remain consistent after deformation. It is therefore necessary, after each deformation iteration, to ensure that all corresponding vertices of the sub-meshes making up the shared boundary are aligned and consistent. This is done by averaging the positions of each corresponding shared boundary vertex, and then updating the shared boundary vertices in the MM2S mesh as well as the sub-meshes with these newly computed vertex positions as in Fig. 3. This process for deforming a multi-material 2-simplex mesh offers many advantages: (1) the proven single surface 2-simplex mesh deformation framework of [1, 2] can be easily utilized, (2) the shared boundary between the sub-meshes will always remain consistent, and (3) there is no need to worry about the non-manifold edges of the shared boundaries since the deformation occurs only on sub-meshes.

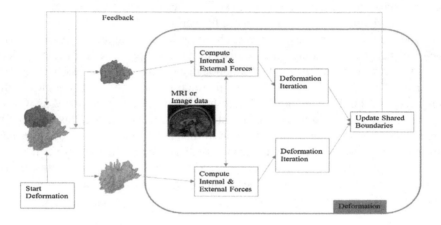

Fig. 3. Overview of the multi-material 2-simplex mesh deformation.

3   Segmenting Structures of the Basal Ganglia

The proposed multi-material 2-simplex deformable system has been also used on realistic data to achieve meaningful segmentation of anatomical structures. The subthalamic nucleus (STN) and the substantia nigra (SN) are two deep brain structures that are difficult to detect and segment from MRI. The proposed system has also been used to segment the globus pallidus (GP), the image gradient of which is better defined. T1-weighted and T2-weighted MR data was used. The MR data used in this section is freely available from Neuroimaging Informatics Tools and Resources Clearinghouse (https://www.nitrc.org/projects/deepbrain7t). A labeled volume is also provided (referred to as the Khan atlas), containing segmentations of the left and right globus pallidus, mammillary body, red nucleus, substantia nigra and subthalamic nucleus. This labeled volume, recently made public, serves as ground truth for validating our multi-surface atlas-to-image registration approach.

3.1 Segmentation of the Subthalamic Nucleus and Substantia Nigra

An initial watertight and 2-manifold multi-material triangular mesh of the left SN-STN was constructed from Chakravarty's atlas [6] using a modified version of the Dual Contouring (DC) algorithm [4]. This atlas has a step size of 0.3 mm, and a triangular mesh generated from this resolution is simply too large (approximately 410 k triangles and 20 k vertices) to be practical. Therefore, the atlas was downsampled to an appropriate size, and a much coarser multi-material triangular mesh was generated (2.5 k triangles and 1.2 k vertices). Figure 4(a) shows a mesh representation of the SN and STN from the Khan atlas, Fig. 4(b) and (c) shows the surface mesh and wireframe mesh, respectively, of the SN and STN constructed using Chakravarty's atlas. For the deformation process, the T2-weighted MR image was used because the SN and STN are more visible than in T1-weighted MR images. The image was anisotropically, and then the gradient image was computed. The external forces for the deformation were computed using the gradient image. Laplacian-based internal forces were used to achieve a smooth mesh. Figure 5 shows the deformation of the SN and STN mesh for several iterations.

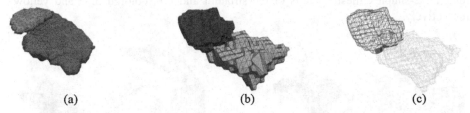

(a) (b) (c)

Fig. 4. (a) A mesh representation of the SN (blue) and STN (pink) from Khan's atlas, (b) the Chakravarty multi-material triangular surface mesh of the SN (yellow) and STN (blue), (c) the wireframe representation of the mesh, where the red part represents the shared boundary. (Color figure online)

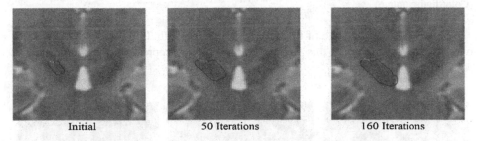

Initial 50 Iterations 160 Iterations

Fig. 5. Deformation of the SN and STN. The red outline represents the outline of the STN and the blue outline represents the outline of the SN. The green outline represents shared boundary. (Color figure online)

3.2 Segmentation of the Globus Pallidus and Striatum

In this section describes an attempt to segment the striatum (comprising the putamen and the caudate nucleus) and the globus pallidus (GP) using high resolution 7 T MR data from [5]. In a T1-weighted MR image, both the striatum and GP have similar intensities, whereas in a T2-weighted MR image the GP appears much more distinct. Both T1 and T2-weighted images are to be used for the deformation process, with the T1-weighted MR image used to mainly drive the deformation of the striatum, and the T2-weighted MR image used to segment the GP. The shared boundary between the striatum and GP will therefore be influenced by both the T1 and T2-weighted images. The main purpose of here is to demonstrate that the proposed multi-material 2-simplex framework can incorporate multi-modal data for deformation. The MR image was anisotropically smoothed, and then the gradient image was computed. Laplacian-based internal forces were used to achieve a smooth mesh.

In order to produce a coarse mesh, the volume was downsampled to an appropriate size and smoothed using a Gaussian blurring-based smoothing process. Our multi-material DC method [4] was then used to create a watertight multi-material triangular surface mesh, which in turn was used by geometric duality to create the initial multi-material 2-simplex mesh. Figure 6 (Left) illustrates the multi-material triangular mesh created by the modified DC algorithm, and Fig. 6 (Right) shows the converted multi-material 2-simplex mesh models of the striatum and GP, colored blue and yellow, respectively.

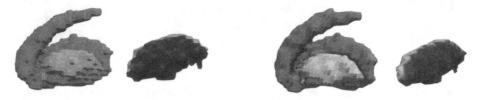

Fig. 6. (Left) The multi-material triangular mesh of the Striatum, colored blue and Globus Pallidus, colored yellow. (Right) The multi-material 2-simplex mesh initialized from the triangular mesh. The red part of the mesh depicts the shared boundary between the GP and St. (Color figure online)

Figure 7 shows the state of the deformation using both T1 and T2-weighted MRI over several iterations. In this figure, the blue outline represents the outline of the

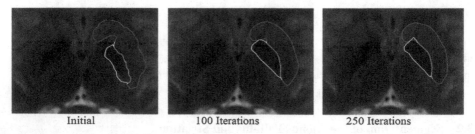

| Initial | 100 Iterations | 250 Iterations |

Fig. 7. Cross-sections of the striatum and globus pallidus during deformation using both T1 and T2-weighted MRI. The blue outline represents the striatum, the yellow outline represents the GP, and the red outline represents the shared boundary. (Color figure online)

striatum, the yellow outline represents the outline of the GP, and the red outline shows the shared boundary between the GP and striatum.

4 Validation

For validation, surface mesh representations of the SN, STN and GP were made from the labeled volume that is a part of the data from [6], and this was used as the ground truth. The opensource VTK libraries implementation of the Marching Cubes algorithm was used to generate the surface meshes. A segmentation of the striatum is not available in the data from [5], and so a quantitative analysis of the striatum is not possible.

The surface-to-surface distance between the deformed mesh and the ground truth mesh of the SN, STN and GP was computed using uniform sampling. The metrics calculated are: Hausdorff Distance (HD), Mean Absolute Distance (MAD), Mean Square Distance (MSD) and Dice's Coefficient (DC), reported in Table 1.

Table 1. Summary of deformation errors. All values in millimeters.

Anatomical structures	HD	MSD	MAD	DC	Max over-segmentation	Max under-segmentation
Subthalamic nucleus	2.1054	0.3087	0.3500	0.7732	1.5529	–0.8978
Substantia nigra	2.5467	0.3578	0.4552	0.7993	1.9724	–1.6345
Globus pallidus	2.4272	0.2166	0.3077	0.9271	2.4272	–2.1850

Figure 8 shows the deformed meshes of the SN, STN and GP. For the deformation of the STN, SN and GP as shown in Fig. 8, the highest over-segmentation error is approximately 1.55 mm, 1.97 mm and 2.42 mm, respectively. The highest under-segmentation error is –0.898 mm, –1.63 mm and –2.19 mm for the STN, SN and GP, respectively.

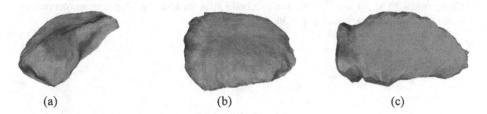

(a)   (b)   (c)

Fig. 8. A color representation of deformation errors for (a) STN, (b) SN and (c) GP. (Color figure online)

Table 1 also shows the HD, MSD, MAD and DC values for the deformed STN, SN and GP. The MSD and MAD values of the STN, SN and GP are smaller because, along the main body of the structures, the segmentation is fairly accurate (as shown by the green coloring in Fig. 8), with over and/or under-segmentation occurring at the lateral ends of the structures, coinciding with lesser gradient values.

5 Conclusion

Accurate representations of anatomical structures in the deep brain regions is very important for medical modelling and simulation purposes. This paper presented a multi-material version of the deformable 2-simplex (MM2S) mesh framework. The meshes are multi-material in the sense that they can have consistent shared boundaries with each other. The MM2S meshes can be generated with relative ease because 2-simplex meshes are topologically dual to triangular meshes. It has been shown that this topological duality can be adapted for converting a multi-material triangular mesh into a multi-material 2-simplex mesh such that the mesh's material information is preserved. The immediate application is ioMRI-ready surgery planning for deep-brain stimulation, however a multi-material deformable surface atlas with shared boundaries is also vital for achieving personalized surface mesh-constrained tetrahedral models for simulation.

References

1. Delingette, H.: General object reconstruction based on simplex meshes. Int. J. Comput. Vis. **32**, 111–146 (1999)
2. Gilles, B., et al.: Musculoskeletal MRI segmentation using multiresolution simplex meshes with medial representations. Med. Image Anal. **14**, 291–302 (2010)
3. Haq, R., Cates, J., Besachio, D.A., Borgie, R.C., Audette, M.A.: Statistical shape model construction of lumbar vertebrae and intervertebral discs in segmentation for discectomy surgery simulation. In: Vrtovec, T., Yao, J., Glocker, B., Klinder, T., Frangi, A., Zheng, G., Li, S. (eds.) CSI 2015. LNCS, vol. 9402, pp. 85–96. Springer, Cham (2016). doi: 10.1007/978-3-319-41827-8_8
4. Rashid, T., Audette, M., et al.: 2-Manifold Surface Meshing Using Dual Contouring with Tetrahedral Decomposition. Adv. Eng. Softw. **106**, 83–96 (2016)
5. Wang, B.T., et al.: Generation and evaluation of an ultra-high-field atlas with applications in DBS planning. In: SPIE Medical Imaging: Image Processing, pp. 97840H–97840H-10 (2016)
6. Chakravarty, M.M., et al.: The creation of a brain atlas for image guided neurosurgery using serial histological data. Neuroimage **30**, 359–376 (2006)

International Workshop
on Point-of-Care Ultrasound:
Algorithms, Hardware,
and Applications, POCUS 2017

Combining Automated Image Analysis with Obstetric Sweeps for Prenatal Ultrasound Imaging in Developing Countries

Thomas L.A. van den Heuvel[1,2]($^{\boxtimes}$), Hezkiel Petros[3], Stefano Santini[3],
Chris L. de Korte[2], and Bram van Ginneken[1,4]

[1] Diagnostic Image Analysis Group, Department of Radiology and Nuclear Medicine,
Radboud University Medical Center, Nijmegen, The Netherlands
[2] Medical Ultrasound Imaging Centre, Department of Radiology and Nuclear
Medicine, Radboud University Medical Center, Nijmegen, The Netherlands
Thomas.vandenHeuvel@radboudumc.nl
[3] St. Luke's Catholic Hospital and College of Nursing and Midwifery,
Wolisso, Ethiopia
[4] Fraunhofer MEVIS, Bremen, Germany

Abstract. Ultrasound imaging can be used to detect maternal risk factors, but it remains out of reach for most pregnant women in developing countries because there is a severe shortage of well-trained sonographers. In this paper we show the potential of combining the obstetric sweep protocol (OSP) with image analysis to automatically obtain information about the fetus. The OSP can be taught to any health care worker without any prior knowledge of ultrasound within a day, obviating the need for a well-trained sonographer to acquire the ultrasound images. The OSP was acquired from 317 pregnant women using a low-cost ultrasound device in St. Luke's Hospital in Wolisso, Ethiopia. A deep learning network was used to automatically detect the fetal head in the OSP data. The fetal head detection was used to detect twins, determine fetal presentation and estimate gestational age without the need of a well-trained sonographer.

Keywords: Prenatal ultrasound · Obstetric sweep protocol · Image analysis

1 Introduction

Worldwide, 99% of all maternal deaths occur in developing countries [1]. Ultrasound imaging can be used to detect risk factors, but requires a well-trained sonographer to obtain and interpret the images. Unfortunately, there is a severe shortage of well-trained sonographers in developing countries [2]. Therefore, ultrasound imaging remains our of reach for most pregnant women in developing countries. In 2011, DeStigter *et al.* introduced the obstetric sweep protocol (OSP) [3]. The OSP consists of six predefined free-hand ultrasound sweeps over

© Springer International Publishing AG 2017
M.J. Cardoso et al. (Eds.): BIVPCS/POCUS 2017, LNCS 10549, pp. 105–112, 2017.
DOI: 10.1007/978-3-319-67552-7_13

the abdomen of the pregnant women, which are visualized in Fig. 1. The main advantage of the OSP is that it can be taught to any health care worker without any prior knowledge of ultrasound within a day, making wide application of this protocol in developing countries feasible. In the paper of DeStiger *et al.* the OSP data was sent via the Internet to radiologists, who interpreted the images and sent back the result to the midwife. In this paper we combine the OSP with image analysis, to automatically detect the fetal head. We show that it is feasible to estimate the gestational age, detect the fetal presentation and detect twin pregnancies with the automated head detection using the OSP data. This would mean that there is no need for a well-trained sonographer to both acquire and interpret the ultrasound images. There is also no need for a technical infrastructure which includes an Internet connection and therefore this represents a next step towards making prenatal ultrasound feasible and accessible to pregnant women in developing countries.

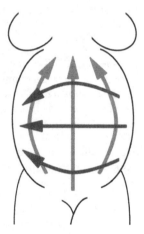

Fig. 1. Visualization of the six free-hand sweeps of the obstetric sweep protocol. The three transverse sweeps are obtained by moving the ultrasound transducer from the pubic bone to the breast bone (green arrows). The three longitudinal sweeps are obtained by moving the ultrasound transducer from the left side of the patient to the right side of the patient (blue arrows). (Color figure online)

2   Methods

2.1   Data

An experienced gynecologist (second author of this paper) acquired both the OSP together with the standard imaging plane, for measuring the reference head circumference (HC), from 317 pregnant women using the MicrUs Ext-1H (Telemed Ultrasound Medical Systems, Italy). The MicrUs EXT-1H is a low-cost ultrasound device which was connected to a mid-range Windows based notebook via USB 3.0. The combination of a low-cost probe and a cheap notebook makes this an affordable and portable solution for obtaining prenatal ultrasound images in developing countries. The data was acquired in St. Luke's Catholic Hospital and College of Nursing and Midwifery in Wolisso, Ethiopia. Acquisition of this data was approved by the local ethics committee.

2.2 Fetal Head Detection

A previously designed deep learning network was used to classify each frame within the OSP data whether the fetal head was present. The deep learning network uses three labels: present, partially present and not present. Present means that the fetal head falls within the field of view (FOV) of the frame. Partially present means that the fetal head falls partially outside of the FOV of the frame, which makes an accurate head circumference measurement impossible. Not present means that the fetal head is not present in the frame. The deep learning network was trained on a separate dataset acquired from 183 pregnant women using the SonoAce R3 (Samsung Medison, Korea). This dataset only contained the three transverse sweeps of the OSP as explained in previous work [4]. The network architecture was inspired by the VGG-Net of Simonyan and Zisserman [5]. The number of deep learning network parameters was minimized, to only 843 thousand parameters, to make deployment on low-cost hardware possible.

2.3 Estimation of Fetal Head Circumference

The OSP data will most likely not contain the standard plane that is normally used to obtain the fetal HC. But in previous work we have shown that it is possible to manually estimate the HC with the use of the OSP data [4]. In this work we used a previously designed CAD system to automatically estimate the HC in a random subset of thirty fetuses (excluding twins), with a GA ranging from 23 until 40 weeks. The CAD system measures the HC in all frames that were classified as containing the fetal head by the deep learning network. The 75th percentile of all measured HCs was taken as the final HC estimation, since the HC obtained in the standard plane is one of the largest circumferences one can measure from a fetal head. The automatically estimated HC was compared to the reference HC, which was obtained by the experience sonographer in the standard plane. The curve of Hadlock [6] was used to determine the GA from the HC.

2.4 Automated Frame Separation

Since the six free-hand sweeps of the OSP were made in a predefined order, it was possible to automatically separate the six sweeps to be able to determine fetal presentation and detect twin pregnancies. The six sweeps were automatically separated using the mean pixel intensity per frame. A threshold was used to determine for which frames the transducer touches the abdomen of the pregnant woman. The threshold is defined by Eq. 1, where μ is the mean frame intensity for all frames of one patient and σ is the standard deviation of the mean intensity per frame.

$$Threshold = \mu - \sigma \tag{1}$$

The largest six connected components were selected as the six sweeps. Smaller connected components were assigned to the nearest sweep. Figure 2 shows the result of the automated frame separation for one patient. This simple procedure turned out to be sufficient for correctly separating the sweeps in 306 of the 317 ultrasound series at our disposal.

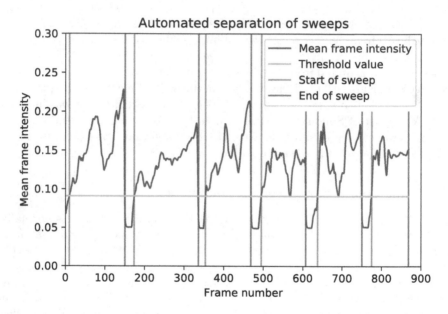

Fig. 2. Visualization of the automated separation of the six sweeps for one patient.

3   Results

Figures 3, 4, and 5 show the result of the fetal head detection by the deep learning network for a fetus in cephalic presentation, a fetus in breech presentation and a twin pregnancy, respectively. The color bar shows the three labels of the network classification. All frames classified as fetal head present (shown in red) were used to automatically estimate the HC. Table 1 shows the mean difference (MD), mean absolute deviation (MAD) and 1.96 standard deviations (SD), between the automatically estimated HC, obtained from the OSP data, and the reference HC, obtained by the experienced gynecologist from the standard imaging plane for the thirty randomly selected cases. The GA could not be computed for six fetuses, because the HC of these fetuses were larger than the largest reported

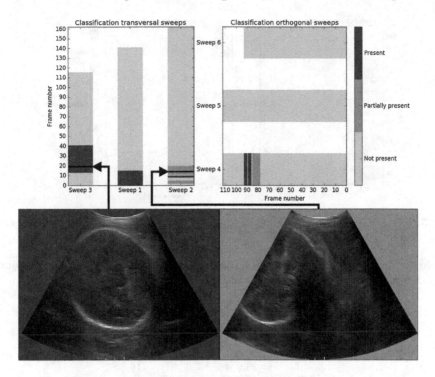

Fig. 3. Visualization of the head detection output by the deep learning network of a fetus in cephalic presentation. The bottom two images show two example frames from the sweep data. The left frame was classified as fetal head present. The right frame was classified as fetal head partially present.

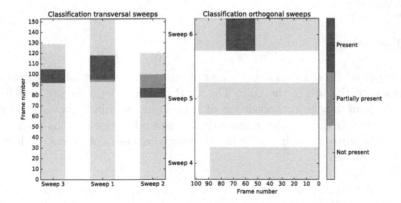

Fig. 4. Visualization of the head detection output by the deep learning network of a fetus in breech presentation.

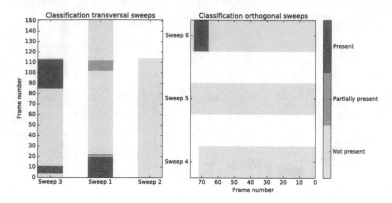

Fig. 5. Visualization of the head detection output by the deep learning network of a twin pregnancy.

Table 1. Mean difference (MD), mean absolute difference (MAD) and 1.96 standard deviations (SD) between the automatic estimation and the manual reference.

	HC (mm)	HC (%)	GA (days)
MD	−6.6[a]	−2.1[a]	−3.6[b]
MAD	11.3[a]	3.7[a]	9.4[b]
1.96 SD	23.9[a]	7.4[a]	16.8[b]

[a]$N = 30$, [b]$N = 24$

value of the curve of Hadlock. This rather high number is associated with the fact that most pregnant women visit the hospital in Ethiopia at a late stage in their pregnancy.

4   Discussion

In this paper we show a system that can automatically extract information about the fetus with the use of the OSP. The OSP can be taught to any health care worker without any prior knowledge of ultrasound within a day. All data for this study were acquired with a low-cost ultrasound device in Ethiopia and the design of the automated image analysis system makes deployment on low-cost hardware possible.

Fetal head detection: The results show that it is possible to automatically detect the fetal head in the OSP frames with the use of the deep learning network. Separation between the head present and partially present was performed to make automated estimation of the HC possible, since the HC can only be measured when the fetal head falls within the FOV of the frame.

Estimation of fetal head circumference: Table 1 shows the MD, MAD and SD between the reference, obtained in the standard plane, and the automated estimation, obtained from the OSP data, for both the HC and GA for thirty randomly selected cases. The literature shows different inter-observer variabilities for the HC measurements. Napolitano *et al.* reported in 2016 an inter-observer variability with a 95% limits of agreement of 4.9% [7], which is only one and a half times smaller compared to our 1.96 SD of 7.4%. Sarris *et al.* reported in 2012 an inter-observer variability with a 1.96 SD of 12.1 mm [8], which is twice as small compared to our 1.96 SD of 23.9 mm, but Sarris *et al.* reported in 2013 a 97th percentile SD of 24.2 mm [9], which very similar to our reported 1.96 SD of 23.9 mm. This comparison shows that the automated system estimates the HC close to the reported inter-observer variability in literature and does this without obtaining the standard imaging plane. The resulting MAD in GA of 9.4 days is very promising for automatic estimation of the GA using the OSP. Future research has to show how this GA estimation can be used in practice.

Determine fetal presentation: Figures 3 and 4 shows that it could be feasible to determine the fetal presentation from the OSP data, making it possible to plan a caesarean section in case of breech presentation. At this moment, the deep learning network only detects the fetal head. Retrain the network to detect both the fetal head and the fetal abdomen could make this method more robust. To the authors knowledge, only Maraci *et al.* have tried to automatically determine fetal presentation with a single free-hand sweep, but this single sweep missed either the fetal head or abdomen in 31% of the 129 test cases [10]. This problem could be solved with the six sweeps of the OSP data, but future work is required to show performance of our approach on the full dataset.

Detecting twin pregnancies: Figure 5 shows the deep learning classification result for a twin pregnancy. Two fetal heads can be discriminated in sweep 1 and 3 of the OSP, so it could be feasible to automatically detect twin pregnancies with the OSP. Future research is required to determine if all 35 twins present in the study data can be detected using the OSP data.

5   Conclusion

This paper shows the feasibility of using prenatal ultrasound in developing countries by combining the obstetric sweep protocol (OSP) with automated image analysis. The OSP can be taught to any health care worker without any prior knowledge of ultrasound within a day, so there is no need for a well-trained sonographer to obtain the ultrasound images. We show that it is feasible to automatically detect basic information about the fetus like: estimation of the gestational age, determine fetal presentation and detect twin pregnancies.

References

1. World Health Organization, UNICEF, UNFPA, The World Bank, the United Nations Population Division: Trends in maternal mortality: 1990 to 2013: estimates by WHO, UNICEF, UNFPA, The World Bank and the United Nations Population Division. World Health Organization (2014)
2. LaGrone, L., Sadasivam, V., Kushner, A., Groen, R.: A review of training opportunities for ultrasonography in low and middle income countries. Trop. Med. Int. Health **17**(7), 808–819 (2012)
3. DeStigter, K.K., Morey, G.E., Garra, B.S., Rielly, M.R., Anderson, M.E., Kawooya, M.G., Matovu, A., Miele, F.R.: Low-cost teleradiology for rural ultrasound. In: Proceedings of the IEEE Global Humanitarian Technology Conference (GHTC), pp. 290–295 (2011)
4. van den Heuvel, T.L.A., Petros, H., Santini, S., de Korte, C.L., van Ginneken, B.: A step towards measuring the fetal head circumference with the use of obstetric ultrasound in a low resource setting. In: SPIE Medical Imaging, vol. 10139, p. 101390V (2017)
5. Simonyan, K., Zisserman, A.: Very deep convolutional networks for large-scale image recognition. arXiv preprint arXiv:1409.1556 (2014)
6. Hadlock, F.P., Harrist, R.B., Sharman, R.S., Deter, R.L., Park, S.K.: Estimation of fetal weight with the use of head, body, and femur measurements-a prospective study. Am. J. Obstet. Gynecol. **151**(3), 333–337 (1985)
7. Napolitano, R., Donadono, V., Ohuma, E.O., Knight, C.L., Wanyonyi, S.Z., Kemp, B., Norris, T., Papageorghiou, A.T.: Scientific basis for standardization of fetal head measurements by ultrasound: a reproducibility study. Ultrasound Obstet. Gynecol. **48**(1), 80–85 (2016)
8. Sarris, I., Ioannou, C., Chamberlain, P., Ohuma, E., Roseman, F., Hoch, L., Altman, D.G., Papageorghiou, A.T.: Intra-and interobserver variability in fetal ultrasound measurements. Ultrasound Obstet. Gynecol. **39**(3), 266–273 (2012)
9. Sarris, I., Ioannou, C., Ohuma, E.O., Altman, D.G., Hoch, L., Cosgrove, C., Fathima, S., Salomon, L.J., Papageorghiou, A.T.: Standardisation and quality control of ultrasound measurements taken in the INTERGROWTH-21st Project. BJOG: Int. J. Obstet. Gynaecol. **120**(s2), 33–37 (2013)
10. Maraci, M.A., Bridge, C.P., Napolitano, R., Papageorghiou, A., Noble, J.A.: A framework for analysis of linear ultrasound videos to detect fetal presentation and heartbeat. Med. Image Anal. **37**, 22–36 (2017)

Automatic Estimation of the Optic Nerve Sheath Diameter from Ultrasound Images

Samuel Gerber[1]([⊠]), Maeliss Jallais[1], Hastings Greer[1], Matt McCormick[1],
Sean Montgomery[2], Bradley Freeman[3], Deborah Kane[3], Deepak Chittajallu[1],
Neal Siekierski[1], and Stephen Aylward[1]

[1] Kitware Inc, Carrboro, NC 27510, USA
samuel.gerber@kitware.com
[2] Duke University, Durham, USA
[3] Washington University, St. Louis, USA

Abstract. We present an algorithm to automatically estimate the diameter of the optic nerve sheath from ocular ultrasound images. The optic nerve sheath diameter provides a proxy for measuring intracranial pressure, a life threating condition frequently associated with head trauma. Early treatment of elevated intracranial pressures greatly improves outcomes and drastically reduces the mortality rate. We demonstrate that the proposed algorithm combined with a portable ultrasound device presents a viable path for early detection of elevated intracranial pressure in remote locations and without access to trained medical imaging experts.

1 Introduction

Portable ultrasound technology is well suited for the development of automated diagnostics systems that enable emergency responders to quickly assess the severity of a patient's injuries. Such light-weight portable automated systems can be employed in remote environments in which expert medical imaging personnel and advanced imaging equipment are not readily available.

This paper considers the application of a point-of-care, computer-assisted ultrasound system for in-field traumatic brain injury (TBI) assessment via the detection of increased intracranial pressure. Delayed treatment of increased intracranial pressure can cause temporary or permanent brain damage or even long-term coma and death. For example, it has been shown that acute subdural hematomas in severe TBI patients cause significant increase in intracranial pressure. Acute subdural hematomas are associated with 90 detected and treated more than 4 h after injury, yet early treatment reduces the mortality rate to 30

In a clinical setting, a non-invasive approach to measure intracranial pressure is by ocular ultrasound. From the ocular ultrasound image the physician manually measures the diameter of optic nerve sheath at a location 3 mm behind the retina. A diameter of the optic nerve greater than 5 mm indicates increased intracranial pressure [Ma2015]. Acquiring such images and making these measurements is a

© Springer International Publishing AG 2017
M.J. Cardoso et al. (Eds.): BIVPCS/POCUS 2017, LNCS 10549, pp. 113–120, 2017.
DOI: 10.1007/978-3-319-67552-7_14

challenging and time consuming task. We propose to automate the process of measuring the diameter of the optic nerve sheath and integrate it with a portable ultrasound system to automatically report elevated intracranial pressure without the need of manually measuring the optic nerve sheath diameter. The ultimate goal is a system that is easy to use and does not require expert personnel or specific training to diagnose TBI.

Using ultrasound for estimation of optic nerve sheath diameter is a well establish approach to diagnose elevated intracranial pressure [Ki2008, Ro2011] and various studies have been performed to establish the optimal threshold for clinical diagnosis [Mo2009, Du2011, Ra2011]. However, to the best of our knowledge this is the first time an algorithm is proposed to automate the estimation process.

2   Algorithm

We propose a two step approach to automate the measurement of the optic nerve sheath diameter. At a high level, the algorithm proceeds by locating the eye through registration of an ellipse with the largest dark circle in the image data. From the ellipse an approximate location of the optic nerve is constructed and used to fit two bars to the walls of the acoustic shadow behind the optic nerve. This high-level description leaves out several intermediate image processing steps, described in detail in Sect. 2.1, that are required to achieve good registration results. Figure 1 shows result of the fitting procedure and illustrates that the proposed algorithm is applicable to a wide variety of ocular ultrasound images.

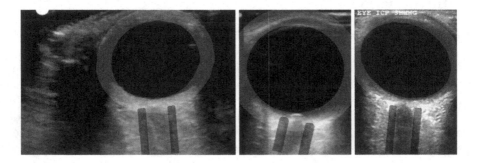

Fig. 1. Result of the proposed algorithm on three ocular ultrasound images. The overlays illustrate the registration results of the algorithm. The blue ellipse delineates the location of they eye and the red bars are the result of fitting the boundary of the acoustic shadow induced by the optic nerve sheath. (Color figure online)

The algorithm is implemented in C++ and is available on github[1]. The user-interface described in Sect. 2.2 is also avaialble on github[2].

---

[1] https://github.com/KitwareMedical/UltrasoundOpticNerveEstimation.
[2] https://github.com/KitwareMedical/UltrasoundIntersonApps.

2.1   Algorithm Details

This section describes the individual image processing steps to achieve an algorithm that performs well on a large variety of images from different types of probes and differences between subjects.

The first part of the algorithm is locating and estimating the size of the eye. The liquid of the vitreous body of the eye has a very low acoustic impedance and appears as black ellipse in B-mode ultrasound images. The boundary of the vitreous body is frequently clearly delineated through the skin of the closed eye and the adjacent tissue. However, acoustic shadows, poor probe contact and collagen floaters cause imperfections in the boundary as well as the interior. Thus, the proposed eye detection algorithm requires several image processing steps illustrated in Fig. 2.

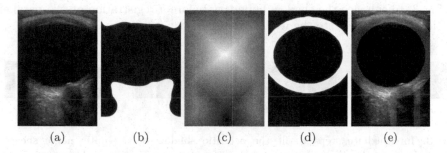

(a)   (b)   (c)   (d)   (e)

Fig. 2. Intermediate steps to locate and estimate the size of the eye. (a) Input image, (b) Gaussian smoothing and threshold, (c) distance transform, (d) the ellipse image generated from the initial eye location and size estimates and (e) the registered ellipse and optic nerve sheath overlayed on the input image.

In detail the steps are:

1. Estimate initial eye center and size:
   (a) Gaussian smoothing, binary thresholding, morphological closing and distance transform.
   (b) The maximum distance provides the initial radius and the location of the maximum distance the initial center of the eye.
2. Refine initial estimates:
   (a) Distance transform over vertical image strip of width 20 pixels around the initial eye center location estimate provides an initial minor ellipse radius.
   (b) Distance transform over horizontal image strip of width 20 pixels around the initial eye center location estimate provides an initial major ellipse radius.
3. Gaussian smoothing and binary thresholding.
4. Create a binary ellipse annulus with the initial estimates of the minor and minor axis of width 0.2 times the major axis with center located at the initial eye center estimate.

5. Register ocular ultrasound (moving image) to ellipse image (fixed image) under an affine transform with a masked mean squared error metric. The mask is an ellipse that encompasses the ellipse annulus on the fixed image. The affine transform is centered on the ellipse center.
6. Refine eye center and major and minor estimates by applying the transform to the minor and major axis vectors and the center point.

The location of they eye provides an approximate region for locating the optic nerve sheath. The optic nerve sheath has a very strong acoustic impedance and reflects a significant amount of the energy of the ultrasound wave. This results in an acoustic shadow that appears as a darker tube behind the optic nerve sheath. We take advantage of this acoustic shadow to estimate the width the optic nerve. The shadow boundary can exhibit several imperfections and have strong intensity variations. We propose several image processing steps, illustrated in Fig. 3, to enhance the shadow boundary before a registration of two parallel vertical bars to delineate the width of the shadow.

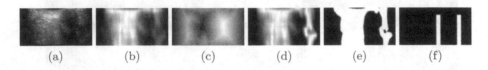

(a)   (b)   (c)   (d)   (e)   (f)

Fig. 3. Intermediate steps to fit the acoustic shadow of the optic nerve sheath. (a) Optic nerve sheath region extract based on the eye location and size estimates, (b) Gaussian smoothing and intensity scaling of individual rows, (c) Distance transform, (d) scaling of rows independently left and right of the initial center (e) thresholding and (f) vertical bars before registration based on initial estimates.

In detail, the optic nerve sheath estimation steps are:

1. Extract optic nerve region below the eye using the eye location and size estimates
2. Gaussian smoothing.
3. Scaling of intensities per individual rows to alleviate attenuation effects.
4. Compute initial center and width estimates:
   (a) Binary threshold, morphological opening and distance transform.
   (b) The maximal distance and its location provide and initial estimate of the optic nerve shadow diameter and its location
5. Scale intensities per row and on each side of the initial optic nerve center estimate independently (Often the left and right boundary exhibit vastly different intensities).
6. Refine initial center and width estimates:
   (a) Binary threshold, morphological opening and distance transform.
7. Use refined center and width to create an image with two vertical bars.

8. Register the two vertical bars (fixed image) to the processed image (moving image) under a similarity transform (rotation, translation and scaling) with a masked mean squared error metric. The mask is a rectangle that encompasses the two vertical bars. The similarity transform is centered on the initial center estimate.
9. Refine width estimates by applying the registration transform to a vector that spans from the left to the right vertical bar of the fixed image.

2.2 Interactive Graphical User Interface

The proposed algorithm is integrated into a user-friendly interface and performs for interactive estimation of the optic nerve sheath diameter. The GUI performs estimates at 4 frames per second, displays the registration results in near real-time and reports statistics of the estimates as they are acquired. Depending on the ultrasound probe, the algorithm can be simplified by skipping the eye estimation step to run at around 20 frames per second. The GUI can be used to report estimates of the optic nerve sheath diameter in near real time as an ultrasound probe is swept across the closed eye of a patient (Fig. 4).

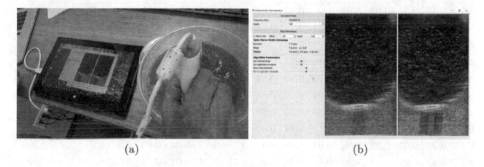

(a)   (b)

Fig. 4. The (a) GUI collecting estimates on an eye phantom in real time and (b) a close-up of the user interface. The GUI is running on a windows tablet connected to a USB linear array ultrasound probe from Interson.

3 Evaluation

We evaluated the performance of the proposed automatic estimator in two ways. In Sect. 3.1 a comparison to manual estimates from novices and medical experts shows that the method has high precision and performs within the range of expert variability. Section 3.2 evaluates the automatic estimates using a gelatine eye phantom with known ground truth diameters and shows that the method is very accurate.

3.1   Comparison to Manual Estimation

For this study 13 volunteers ranging from novices to medical professionals annotated 23 ocular ultrasound images from the internet (in pixel units due to unknown image spacing units). Two linear regressions of the automatic estimates with two different parameter settings against the estimates of a medical expert resulted in an R^2 of 0.82 and 0.91, respectively. Both linear regressions were statistically significant with a p-value on the order of machine precision ($2e^{-16}$).

Table 1 contains all pairwise correlations between all participants of the study as well as two automatic estimates with different parameter settings.

Table 1. Pairwise Pearson's correlation coefficients between novice (N1 - N10), expert (E1 - E3) and automatic (A1, A2) estimates.

	N1	N2	N3	N4	N5	N6	N7	N8	N9	N10	E1	E2	E3	A1	A2
N1	1	0.42	0.34	0.29	0.33	0.68	0.32	0.91	0.56	0.29	0.52	0.54	0.36	0.35	0.52
N2	0.42	1	0.83	0.93	0.92	0.85	0.95	0.56	0.83	0.93	0.86	0.91	0.95	0.91	0.89
N3	0.34	0.83	1	0.88	0.92	0.84	0.90	0.45	0.70	0.91	0.80	0.74	0.88	0.83	0.83
N4	0.29	0.93	0.88	1	0.94	0.80	0.96	0.42	0.74	0.97	0.82	0.83	0.94	0.92	0.85
N5	0.33	0.92	0.92	0.94	1	0.83	0.93	0.45	0.72	0.94	0.83	0.82	0.91	0.85	0.85
N6	0.68	0.85	0.84	0.80	0.83	1	0.83	0.75	0.79	0.82	0.83	0.84	0.83	0.83	0.86
N7	0.32	0.95	0.90	0.96	0.93	0.83	1	0.46	0.83	0.95	0.80	0.90	0.97	0.95	0.89
N8	0.91	0.56	0.45	0.42	0.45	0.75	0.46	1	0.60	0.45	0.60	0.66	0.51	0.51	0.63
N9	0.56	0.83	0.70	0.74	0.72	0.79	0.83	0.60	1	0.73	0.82	0.88	0.82	0.74	0.78
N10	0.29	0.93	0.91	0.97	0.94	0.82	0.95	0.45	0.73	1	0.85	0.80	0.94	0.91	0.84
E1	0.52	0.86	0.80	0.82	0.83	0.83	0.80	0.60	0.82	0.85	1	0.71	0.82	0.72	0.77
E2	0.54	0.91	0.74	0.83	0.82	0.84	0.90	0.66	0.88	0.80	0.71	1	0.90	0.88	0.87
E3	0.36	0.95	0.88	0.94	0.91	0.83	0.97	0.51	0.82	0.94	0.82	0.90	1	0.95	0.90
A1	0.35	0.91	0.83	0.92	0.85	0.83	0.95	0.51	0.74	0.91	0.72	0.88	0.95	1	0.92
A2	0.52	0.89	0.83	0.85	0.85	0.86	0.89	0.63	0.78	0.84	0.77	0.87	0.90	0.92	1

Table 2 provides a summary of the pairwise correlations and reports the intra- and inter-correlation between novice, expert and automatic estimates. The estimates from the novice N1 were far off from any of the other novices and was excluded from the results reported in Tabel 2. The automatic estimates are more strongly correlated (0.85) to the medical expert than the correlation within the group of medical experts (0.81).The correlation among experts matches results of previous studies [Ze2014, Jo2016]. Thus, the proposed automatic estimator performs on par or even better than the medical experts.

3.2   Gel Phantom Study

This evaluation is based on an eye phantom using 3D-printed optic nerves (plastic discs) of known diameter embedded under gelatine orbs as described in detail

Table 2. Inter- and intra-correlations (mean Pearson correlation coefficients) among novice (excluding N1), expert and automated estimates.

	Novice	Expert	Automatic
Novice	0.78	0.83	0.82
Expert	0.83	0.81	0.85
Automatic	0.82	0.85	0.92

in [Ze2014]. The eye phantom produces ultrasound images that closely resemble clinical ocular ultrasound images.

The goal of this evaluation is to check if an accurate estimate of the optic nerve is possible with the proposed algorithm. We imaged the phantom using the graphical user interface described in Sect. 2.2 connected to an Interson linear array probe with 127 transducer elements and a pixel resolution of 0.8 mm. A novice (non-medical imaging expert) used the graphical user-interface, which shows B-mode images in real-time, to first locate the optic nerve. Once the probe was positioned to deliver a good image of the optic nerve, as judged by the novice user, the automatic estimation process was started and run interactively for about 10 s. This resulted in approximately 40 to 50 optic nerve sheath diameter estimates.

Table 3 shows that, in this controlled setting, the means of the automatic estimates are within less than +/- 5 mm and a relatively tight distribution of estimates around the ground truth diameter.

Table 3. Automatic estimation results on eye phantom.

Disc size	Mean	Std. deviation	Low. quartile	Median	Up. quartile
7 mm	7 mm	1 mm	6.4 mm	6.9 mm	7.7 mm
6 mm	6.1 mm	1 mm	5.8 mm	6.4 mm	6.6 mm
5 mm	5.1 mm	1.4 mm	4.4 mm	4.9 mm	5.7 mm
4 mm	4.4 mm	0.6 mm	4.2 mm	4.3 mm	4.5 mm
3 mm	3.4 mm	1.1 mm	2.9 mm	3.2 mm	3.5 mm

The standard deviations of the individual measurements per disc are too large to accurately suggest elevated intracranial pressure. However, the mean deviation of the mean estimates from the ground truth over the 5 measurements is only 0.2 mm with a standard deviation of 0.18 mm. This suggest that the means reported by the automatic estimation procedure measurements are accurate enough to determine elevated intracranial pressure. In this small study the proposed algorithm yields more accurate results than reported in a study on intra-operator variations of manual estimates on the same type of phantom, but with higher resolution ultrasound probes, reports an average bias of 0.33 mm and standard deviations of 0.64 mm of the measurements [Jo2016].

4   Conclusion

The results presented indicate that the algorithm performs well in a controlled setting. A retrospective analysis of clinical images indicates that our system performs similar to an expert, and a phantom study using 3D printed optic nerves of known diameter suggests that our system is accurate.

The next step is to automatically identify high quality images as a probe is swept over the eye. This will eliminate the need for the operator to view, interpret, or make measurements on an ultrasound image when using it to assess a dilated optic nerve sheath. Ultimately, we aim for a system that can be used by novice operators with minimal ultrasound experience. The system will report when a sufficient number of high quality images have been acquired for an accurate estimate of the diameter. Based on this estimate it will be able to automatically indicate if the diameter of the optic nerve is greater than 5 mm and alert the user elevated intracranial pressure.

The long term goal is to develop a lightweight portable ultrasound system that, in addition to automated diagnosis of TBI, includes automatic diagnosis tools for pneumothorax (detached lung) and internal bleeding.

This work was supported, in part, by NIH/NIBIB and NIH/NIGMS via 1R01EB021396-01A1: Slicer+PLUS: Point-of-Care Ultrasound.

References

Du2011. Dubourg, J., et al.: Ultrasonography of optic nerve sheath diameter for detection of raised intracranial pressure: a systematic review and meta-analysis. Intensive Care Med. **37**(7), 1059–1068 (2011)

Jo2016. Johnson, G.R.J., et al.: Estimating the accuracy of optic nerve sheathdiameter measurement using a pocket-sized, handheld ultrasound on a simulation model. Crit. Ultrasound J. **8**(1), 18 (2016)

Ki2008. Kimberly, H.H., et al.: Correlation of optic nerve sheath diameter with direct measurement of intracranial pressure. Acad. Emerg. Med. **15**(2), 201–204 (2008)

Ma2015. Maissan, I.M., Dirven, P.J., Haitsma, I.K., Hoeks, S.E., Gommers, D., Stolker, R.J.: Ultrasonographic measured optic nerve sheath diameter as an accurate and quick monitor for changes in intracranial pressure. J. Neurosurg. **123**(3), 37–74 (2015)

Mo2009. Moretti, R., et al.: Reliability of optic nerve ultrasound for the evaluation of patients with spontaneous intracranial hemorrhage. Neurocrit. Care **11**(3), 406 (2009)

Ra2011. Rajajee, V., et al.: Optic nerve ultrasound for the detection of raised intracranial pressure. Neurocrit. Care **15**(3), 506–515 (2011)

Ro2011. Rosenberg, J.B., et al.: Non-invasive methods of estimating intracranial pressure. Neurocrit. Care **15**(3), 599–608 (2011)

Se1981. Seelig, J.M., et al.: Traumatic acute subdural hematoma: major mortality reduction in comatose patients treated within four hours. N. Engl. J. Med. **304**(25), 1511–1518 (1981)

Ze2014. Zeiler, F.A., et al.: A unique model for ONSD Part II: inter/intra-operator variability. Can. J. Neurol. Sci. **41**, 430–435 (2014)

Achieving Fluid Detection by Exploiting Shadow Detection Methods

Matthias Noll[1,2]([✉]), Julian Puhl[1], and Stefan Wesarg[1]

[1] Visual Healthcare Technologies, Fraunhofer IGD, Darmstadt, Germany
{matthias.noll,julian.puhl,stefan.wesarg}@igd.fraunhofer.de
[2] GRIS, Technische Universität Darmstadt, Darmstadt, Germany
http://s.fhg.de/vht

Abstract. Ultrasound provides a useful and readily available imaging tool. The big challenge in acquiring a good ultrasound image are possible shadow artefacts that hide anatomical structures. This applies in particular to 3D ultrasound acquisitions, because shadow artefacts may be recorded outside the visualized image plane. There are only a few automatic methods for shadow artefact detection. In our work we like to introduce a new shadow detection method that is based on an adaptive thresholding approach. The development was attempted, after existing methods had been extended to separate shadow and fluid regions. The entire detection procedure utilizes only the ultrasound scan line information and some basic knowledge about the ultrasound propagation inside the human body. Applying our method, the ultrasound operator can retrieve combined information about shadow and fluid locations, that may be invaluable for image acquisition or diagnosis. The method can be applied to conventional 2D as well as 3D ultrasound images.

Keywords: Ultrasound · Shadow artefact · Free fluid · Detection

1 Introduction

Ultrasound shadows are a big challenge in ultrasound imaging. This is especially true when applying 3D ultrasound, because there is only a finite number of image planes that can be simultaneously visualized to the operator in a meaningful way. Important secondary structures that are off screen might be hidden inside a shadow artefact without the ultrasound operator even noticing. Automatic detection methods for ultrasound shadows can help to minimize shadow recording by indicating their presence during or after the acquisition. However, shadow detection methods have not been a great focus in the literature. A possible reason for that is, that shadows can be easily spotted in conventional 2D images, which are still the clinical standard. However, 3D ultrasound continues to be applied more often, but herein shadows can't be spotted as easily. In our work we like to provide tools that enable the shadow detection and allow for better image acquisitions. Besides shadows, fluids are also displayed with dark

© Springer International Publishing AG 2017
M.J. Cardoso et al. (Eds.): BIVPCS/POCUS 2017, LNCS 10549, pp. 121–128, 2017.
DOI: 10.1007/978-3-319-67552-7_15

intensity values in the B-mode image. A general separation of both would be ideal to allow further diagnosis potential. Especially for trauma and acitis patients, a combined free fluid and shadow detection would assist the physician. In the next sections we provide some information about existing literature approaches. In our work we have enhances one of those methods to additionally achieve free fluid separation from shadow regions. The approach was then altered to allow a more simple thresholding based separation of shadows and fluids from normal tissue. The achievable result may be exploited in automatic image analysis methods.

2   Shadow and Fluid Detection

To better understand the concept of our shadow and fluid detection method, we give a brief overview on how the B-mode ultrasound image is generated. The ultrasound transducer emits the ultrasound signal into the body. While passing through the different tissue layers, the signal is attenuated due to reflection, absorption and scattering of the ultrasound signal. The B-mode image is generated from the reflected signals by evaluating both the signal strength and the signal run-time. The former determines the grey value and the latter determines the depth along the ultrasound propagation direction. The inherent ultrasound speckle noise is the result of the signal scattering at the tissue structures.

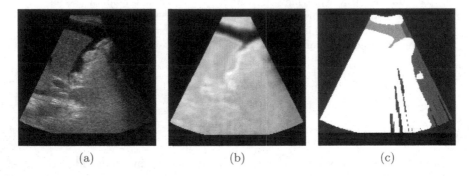

(a)   (b)   (c)

Fig. 1. Illustration of the shadow detection method in [6], with the B-mode input (a), the entropy feature image (b), the detected shadow (dark grey) as well as the fluid detection enhancement (light grey) (c).

Ultrasound shadows and fluids are both mapped to dark B-mode intensity values. Shadows are dark because most of the ultrasound signal is reflected at some point along the ultrasound propagation direction. This prevents the ultrasound signal from reaching deeper tissue layers and generates the characteristic posterior shadow artefact. The reflections are caused by a significant change in the tissue impedance which occurs among others at bone structures. Fluids appear dark, because there are only small reflections within the fluid region that exhibit a low signal strength. As a result, the ultrasound signal at the end of the fluid region is approximately as strong as it was at the its beginning.

Only a few methods for both fluid and shadow detection have been presented in the literature. A threshold based approach for free fluid segmentation has been introduced in [3]. The method utilizes the accumulated intensity difference of a pixels eight neighborhood to classify it as part of a fluid region or not. Other publications like [4] or [2,6] have presented methods to detect ultrasound shadows. In [4] the authors determine the probability, that a signal transmitted from each pixel location can reach the transducer receiver. To achieve this all neighboring pixels are connect to a pixel network with high intensity pixels serving as attenuating network nodes. The signal simulation is performed using a random walker approach. Both latter methods [2,6] utilize simulated scan lines along the ultrasound propagation direction to detect signal discontinuities that correspond to shadow interfaces. Also, both methods use the local Shannon entropy as the detection feature (c.f. Fig. 1).

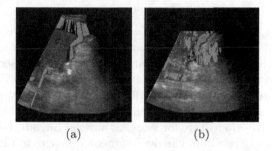

(a)   (b)

Fig. 2. Illustration of a promising new fluid feature, that is generated along simulated scan lines. The feature represents sections along scan lines with a similar intensity value at the section start and end. Two feature examples are given in (a) and (b), with (b) being slightly oversegmented.

To achieve free fluid as well as shadow detection, we have extended the shadow detection method in [6] so that it generates additional fluid entries to the methods confidence mask. The basis of our approach is, that fluids are usually surrounded by tissue structures that hold them. On this account, tissue layers with higher intensities should exist below the darker fluid region. Shadows on the other hand do not permit the existence of such layers. A shadow always continues as far as the bottom of the ultrasound image. Thus, a fluid region may be detected along a scan line as a scan line section, if a sufficiently large or high valued tissue region lies adjacent to the fluid section. We have implemented this premise as a basic threshold t_r for the remaining scan line pixels after the potential fluid section. We have noticed, that for an easy application of the threshold, a backward accumulation of the scan line intensities is preferable to the original approach. This way, the remaining scan line energy can be directly accessed as a scan line entry. The result of our enhancement is given as an example in Fig. 1c, with tissue (white; 255), fluid (light grey; 127) and shadow (dark grey; 64) pixels determined along the scan lines. Because the approach utilizes the image entropy for the detection (c.f. Fig. 1b), the branch in the newly detected fluid region is swallowed up by the blurred tissue edges.

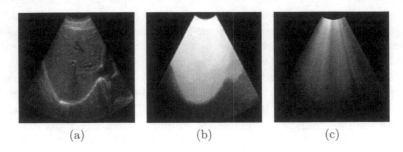

(a)   (b)   (c)

Fig. 3. The backwards accumulation result (c) compared to the results (b) of the shadow detection in [4], with (a) being the input image.

To correct this, we have attempted to extract the fluid region directly by establishing a fluid feature, that is characterized by the earlier mentioned properties. The basic idea to generate the feature is, to search for sections along the scan line, that show only a slight increase in intensity, while at the same time having approximately the same intensities at the sections' start and end. We achieve this by backtracking the pixel intensities along the scan line. The approach is not unlike the dip feature for vessels, that was introduced in [7]. In Fig. 2 we provide a promising result and an oversegmented image. In Fig. 2a the feature does not fully cover the entire fluid region. Also in Fig. 2b it also responds in the tissue region, which is sufficiently dark and mistaken as fluid. Further research is necessary to improvement the feature. The goal is to highlighting the entire fluid region and reducing the amount of included tissue sections.

Furthermore, due to the alteration of the methods accumulation direction to a backward accumulation, we now generate an image that is comparable to the results of the method in [4] (see Fig. 3c and Fig. 3b). Both images show the tissue area of a liver, though not generated on the same image. Dark image regions denote the possible existence of shadowing. The mask can be used to separate tissue from shadows and the background, as can be seen in Fig. 4. The tissue mask (Fig. 4b) was generated using a simple threshold. The shadow mask (Fig. 4c) is derived as the inverted tissue mask.

Because both target regions (fluid and shadows) mostly consist of dark intensities, a well defined threshold t_s should be sufficient to separate the target from tissue information. The challenge is, that ultrasound intensities are in no way normalized and can vary strongly between ultrasound devices. Also, fluids and shadow intensities are not always as dark as one would suspect. A threshold should be able to adapt to this difference in data.

Thus, our proposed algorithm aims to achieve the same results as the enhanced method in Fig. 1c. But instead of using an entropy criterion to detect

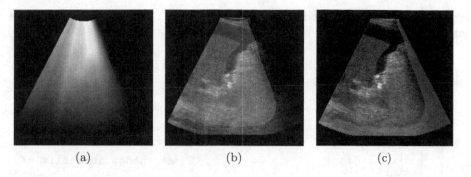

(a)   (b)   (c)

Fig. 4. The intensities accumulated backwards (from the bottom to the top) (a), the thresholded tissue masks (b) and its inversion, the shadow mask (c).

and evaluate discontinuities along scan lines, we like to extract the target regions by only applying good thresholds and perform a pixelwise classification. The basis for the approach is a denoised image. The noise reduction is necessary, because we do not want speckle and other artefacts to have a huge impact on the classification result. Most methods utilize speckle reduction methods that are based on different statistical distribution models like Rayleigh or Fisher-Tippett [5]. Another way of reducing speckle is the nonlinear, so called total variation (TV) filtering. The TV filter tries to reconstruct the "original" signal from the available data, by minimization of the global total variational (L^1) [1]. The filter can achieve this even at low signal-to-noise ratios, which ultrasound is known for. The optimization problem is solved iteratively and does reduce noise while simultaneously preserving edges.

We propose our algorithm as follows: On the smoothed image, we first determine the maximum (i_{max}) and minimum (i_{min}) pixel intensities to initialize the adaptive threshold value g for the fluid and shadow regions. The threshold g is calculated as

$$g = i_{min} + (i_{max} - i_{min}) * \lambda \tag{1}$$

The factor λ can be used to adjust the threshold location further, e.g. through a user interaction. The default value for λ was chosen as $1/8$ because it is sufficiently dark and worked best on the test images. For the detection we simulate scan lines for 3D or 2D images as in [6] and [2]. Applying the calculated threshold g on the input image, all remaining intensities are accumulated along the simulated scan lines. As a result we obtain the thresholded accumulation image I_{e_g}.

Given that the pixel intensity is equal to the energy that was reflected at some image location, the last value of each scan line holds the total energy $e_{i_{max}}$ that was reflected by the tissue pixels along that scan line. This value is transferred to each entry of the sampled scan line positions, which produces the maximum energy image $I_{e_{max}}$.

To generate the threshold based detection result of shadows and fluids, we apply Algorithm 1. The algorithm iterates over the entire image I and classifies each pixels affiliation to one of the target regions based on the difference in accumulated threshold intensities g. Function $f(p, I)$ extracts the intensity of pixel p from the given image I.

Data: $I_{e_{max}}$, I_{e_g} and g
Result: confidence mask with fluids, shadow and tissue regions
for *each pixel $p_i \in I$* **do**
    if $f(p_i, I) < g$ **then**
        if $f(p_i, I_{e_{max}}) - f(p_i, I_{e_g}) > m \cdot \gamma$ **then**
            $p_i = 127$;   /* fluid intensity */
        else
            $p_i = 64$;   /* shadow intensity */
        end
    end
end

Algorithm 1. Separation of fluid and shadow pixels.

3   Results and Evaluation

A qualitative comparison between the original algorithm, including the enhancements for fluid detection (5b), and the new threshold based approach (5c) is given in Fig. 5. The result of the thresholding approach basically shows the same fluid and shadow regions as the original algorithm. However, due to the pixelwise classification, the result looks smoother and exhibits less tearing in form of faulty shadow detection, as can be seen in the bottom center. Furthermore, the fluid region could be extended to include most of the downwards oriented fluid branch, that was not detected in the modification of the original algorithm, due to the diffused entropy image (c.f. Fig. 1b). Additional results that show a variety of image types are provided in Fig. 7.

Our threshold method results were compared to the algorithms in [2,6] with the method in [2] being ported to 3D. The results can be seen in Table 1. The

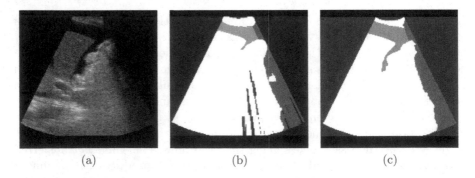

(a)   (b)   (c)

Fig. 5. A comparisson of the original entropy based algorithm including the added fluid detection extension (b) and the new threshold based detection approach (c), with (a) being the input image.

Table 1. Ground truth evaluation of the proposed method.

	[2] ∅	[6] ∅	proposed method ∅
DICE Coefficient	0,8915	0,9050	0,902012
Relative Absolute Volume Difference[%]	18.3091	-0.6448	-13,26295

DICE coefficient for the proposed method is approximately the same as in [6]. However, the relative absolute volume difference deviates to the negative. This is due to the parameter γ, since it can be chosen to adapt the result. At the default setting with $\gamma = 1/8$, the algorithm is more conservative in extending the tissue region, so more pixels are classified as shadows.

Because we currently apply the total variation filtering, the processing speed is quite slow. The TV filtering at 20 iterations alone requires approximately 60% of the algorithms processing time. A 3D volume is processed in 12-15 s. The 2D processing can be performed in 1600 ms, while the noise removal requires roughly 1040 ms. Though, no optimizations have been attempted so far.

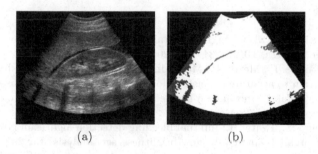

(a)   (b)

Fig. 6. Free fluid detection in Morison's pouch, between liver and kidney (b) applying the new algorithm (a). source: wikipedia.org

4   Discussion

We have extended a literature shadow detection method to simultaneously detect shadows and free fluid regions (see Fig. 6.). The detection result was introduced to the output label map as an additional fluid label. The method was then further adapted to only require adaptive thresholds, that can be derived from the image content. Those have replaced the entropy feature along scan lines of the original approach. The output map can help the operator to collect images with less shadowing while also classifying the image content. Because of the fluid and shadow separation, the map can also be helpful for trauma scenarios as well as acitis cases. We have briefly introduced a new fluid feature that might be useful in different future scenarios. Further development should focus on enhancing the algorithm speed and optimization of the parameter γ.

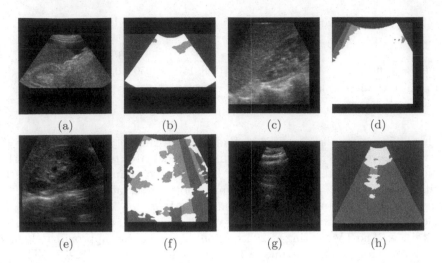

(a)   (b)   (c)   (d)

(e)   (f)   (g)   (h)

Fig. 7. Additional results of the threshold based shadow and fluid detection algorithm.

References

1. Chan, T., Osher, S., Shen, J.: The digital tv filter and nonlinear denoising. IEEE Trans. Image Process. **10**(2), 231–241 (2001)
2. Hellier, P., Coupe, P., Meyer, P., Morandi, X., Collins, D.: Acoustic shadows detection, application to accurate reconstruction of 3d intraoperative ultrasound. In: 5th IEEE International Symposium on Biomedical Imaging: From Nano to Macro, 2008, ISBI 2008, pp. 1569–1572, May 2008
3. Ito, K., Sugano, S., Iwata, H.: Internal bleeding detection algorithm based on determination of organ boundary by low-brightness set analysis. In: 2012 IEEE/RSJ International Conference on Intelligent Robots and Systems (IROS), pp. 4131–4136, October 2012
4. Karamalis, A., Wein, W., Klein, T., Navab, N.: Ultrasound confidence maps using random walks. Med. Image Anal. **16**(6), 1101–1112 (2012). http://www.science direct.com/science/article/pii/S1361841512000977
5. Michailovich, O.V., Tannenbaum, A.: Despeckling of medical ultrasound images. IEEE Trans. Ultrason. Ferroelectr. Freq. Control **53**(1), 64–78 (2006). http://www. ncbi.nlm.nih.gov/pmc/articles/PMC3639001/
6. Noll, M., Puhl, J., Wesarg, S.: Enhanced shadow detection for 3D ultrasound. In: Deserno, T.M., Handels, H., Meinzer, H.-P., Tolxdorff, T. (eds.) Bildverarbeitung für die Medizin 2014. I, pp. 234–239. Springer, Heidelberg (2014). doi:10.1007/ 978-3-642-54111-7_45
7. Penney, G., Blackall, J., Hamady, M., Sabharwal, T., Adam, A., Hawkes, D.: Registration of freehand 3d ultrasound and magnetic resonance liver images. Med. Image Anal. **8**(1), 81–91 (2004). http://view.ncbi.nlm.nih.gov/pubmed/14644148

A Probe-Camera System for 3D Ultrasound Image Reconstruction

Koichi Ito[1(✉)], Kouya Yodokawa[1], Takafumi Aoki[1], Jun Ohmiya[2],
and Satoshi Kondo[2]

[1] Graduate School of Information Sciences, Tohoku University,
6-6-05, Aramaki Aza Aoba, Sendai 980-8579, Japan
`ito@aoki.ecei.tohoku.ac.jp`
[2] Konica Minolta, Inc., 12, Sakura Machi, Takatsuki 569-8503, Japan

Abstract. This paper proposes a probe-camera system for 3D ultrasound (US) image reconstruction with probe-camera calibration and probe localization methods. The probe-camera calibration method employs an existing US phantom for convenience with a simple procedure. The probe localization method employs structure from motion (SfM) to estimate the camera motion. SfM is used to reconstruct 3D point clouds from multiple-view images and simultaneously estimate each camera position. Through experiments using the developed system, we demonstrate that the proposed method exhibits good performance to reconstruct 3D US volume.

Keywords: 3D ultrasound · Probe localization · Structure from motion

1 Introduction

Ultrasound imaging has three key advantages: (i) high spatial resolution, (ii) real-time imaging and (iii) non-invasiveness. US imaging is useful in point-of-care due to such key advantages. Recently, three-dimensional (3D) US has attracted much attention as a valuable imaging tool for a diagnostic procedure. This paper explores 3D US imaging in the point of care. 3D US is acquired by sweeping a US probe around the area of interests and integrating a set of US images to reconstruct 3D volume data. Among 3D US acquisition protocols, we focus on the freehand protocol [2] because of its cost-effectiveness and flexibility. The quality of 3D volume data significantly depends on the accuracy of probe localization.

There are some approaches to estimate the motion of US probes. The first approach is to use electromagnetic (EM) device to know the accurate position of US probes [5,13]. The accuracy of probe localization is high, while the special devices are required resulting in increasing cost. EM devices also have to be attached on the US probe resulting in interfering the smooth manipulation and EM devices are sensitive to ferromagnetic materials. The second approach is to use an optical tracker to measure the position of US probes [3,15]. The accuracy of probe localization is relatively high, while the optical sensors are required

© Springer International Publishing AG 2017
M.J. Cardoso et al. (Eds.): BIVPCS/POCUS 2017, LNCS 10549, pp. 129–137, 2017.
DOI: 10.1007/978-3-319-67552-7_16

resulting in increasing cost. The third approach is to use markers to estimate the motion of US probes [6,10,12]. The motion of the US probe is estimated by detecting markers from the captured video sequence. The cost of the system is cheaper than the first and second approaches, since only a camera is required, while markers must be attached on the skin surface, resulting in decreasing the flexibility and acceptability.

Sun et al. [16] proposed a markerless freehand 3D US method. The motion of the US probe is estimated only from a video sequence of skin patterns captured by a low-cost camera using simultaneous localization and mapping (SLAM). This method is cost-effective compared with other methods, but the accuracy has to be improved, since the cumulative estimation error of the probe motion is about 10 mm for the probe travel distance of 100 mm. Ito et al. [8] proposed a 3D US imaging method using structure from motion (SfM). SfM [4,17] is one of 3D reconstruction methods in the field of computer vision and is used to reconstruct the sparse 3D point clouds from multiple-view images and simultaneously estimate each camera position. To apply SfM to a video sequence, an accurate method is required to track features between adjacent frames. The motion estimation error is about 2 mm for the probe travel distance of 200 mm.

The above methods [8,16] need the geometric relationship between the US probe and the camera so as to estimate the accurate US probe motion. Sun et al. [16] manually measured the position of the US probe and the camera. Ito et al. [8] assumed the translational displacement of the US probe and the camera. In practice, there is a complex movement of the US probe, since the human body consists of soft, curved and complex structures. Calibration between the US probe and the camera is indispensable for reconstructing accurate 3D US volume data. To address the above problem, this paper develops an Ultrasound Probe-Camera System (UPCS) for reconstructing 3D volume data and proposes a calibration method for UPCS. Through experiments using the developed UPCS, we demonstrate that the proposed method exhibits good performance to reconstruct 3D US volume.

2   US Probe-Camera System (UPCS)

UPCS consists of an ultrasound diagnostic system and a camera. US images are acquired by SONIMAGE HS1 (Konica Minolta, Inc.) with L18-4 linear probe (center frequency: 10 MHz) as shown in Fig. 1(a), where the field of view (FOV) of US images is 40×38 mm, the frame rate is 30 fps and the recording time is 10 seconds, i.e., 300 frames. A camera is C920 (Logicool, Webcam C920), where the image size is 640×480 pixels and the frame rate is 30 fps. The camera is attached on the US probe as shown in Fig. 1(b).

3   US Probe-Camera Calibration

This section describes the proposed calibration method between the US probe and the camera. Figure 2(a) shows a flow diagram of the proposed calibration method.

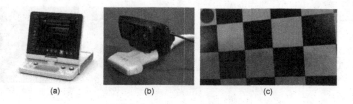

Fig. 1. Developed UPCS for 3D US volume reconstruction: (a) US diagnostic system, (b) camera attached on a US probe and (c) checker pattern used for camera calibration.

First, camera calibration is performed to obtain the intrinsic parameters of the camera, i.e., focal length, image center and lens distortion. We employ the camera calibration toolbox for MATLAB[1]. Next, probe localization is performed using the US phantom, which is used to evaluate the spatial resolution, contrast, and geometry of the US probe. Figure 2(b) shows the US phantom used in the experiment, RMI 403GS LE (Gammex, Inc.). This phantom is filled with water-based gels with the appearance of human tissue and includes 8 nylon wires of 0.1 mm in diameter with a 2 cm interval. The US probe is located perpendicular to the horizontal plane of the phantom so that 8 wires are on the straight line as shown in Fig. 2(c). Then, the extrinsic parameters, i.e., rotation R and translation t, are estimated. Correspondence between the US probe and the camera cannot be used for calibration, since the US probe observes the inside of the phantom, while the camera observes the surface of the phantom. We estimate the geometric relationship between the camera and the checker pattern and between the US probe and the checker pattern, putting a checker pattern on the surface of the phantom.

We assume that the center of the probe coordinate system is the center of the contact area between the US probe and the phantom. Let one of corner points of the checker pattern be the center of the world coordinate system, M_w. The rotation matrix R_p and the translation vector t_p from the probe center to M_w are estimated. Note that R_p is an identity matrix, since the US probe is located perpendicular to the horizontal plane of the phantom as mentioned above. Hence, all we have to do is to measure the translational displacement t_p between the probe center to M_w. The rotation matrix R_c and t_c from the camera center to M_w can be estimated using the same approach of camera calibration.

The geometric relationship between 3D point M_c in the camera coordinate system and 3D point M_p in the probe coordinate system is defined by

$$M_c = R_c M_w + t_c, \tag{1}$$
$$M_p = R_p M_w + t_p. \tag{2}$$

---

[1] Camera Calibration Toolbox for MATLAB: http://www.vision.caltech.edu/bouguetj/calib_doc/.

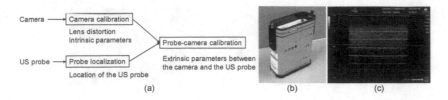

Fig. 2. Calibration between the US probe and the camera: (a) flow diagram of probe-camera calibration, (b) phantom used in the calibration and (c) US image of the phantom.

Equation (1) is modified as

$$M_w = R_c^T M_c - R_c^T t_c. \tag{3}$$

Substituting this equation into Eq. (2), we obtain

$$M_p = R_p R_c^T M_c - R_p R_c^T t_c + t_p \tag{4}$$

$$= R M_c + t, \tag{5}$$

where $R = R_p R_c^T$ and $t = -R_p R_c^T t_c + t_p$. The camera motion can be converted into the probe motion using Eq. (5). Note that Eq. (5) can be derived by estimating only the extrinsic parameter of the camera, if the probe center is set to M_w.

4   3D US Volume Reconstruction

This section describes 3D US volume reconstruction from a US video sequence. This paper employs the similar method proposed by Ito et al. [8]. Figure 3 shows a flow diagram of the proposed method, which consists of 5 steps: (i) contrast enhancement, (ii) feature point tracking, (iii) Structure from Motion (SfM), (iv) coordinate conversion and (v) 3D reconstruction. The following is the brief description for each step.

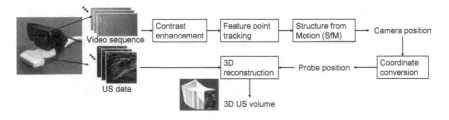

Fig. 3. Flow diagram of 3D US volume reconstruction.

4.1   Contrast Enhancement

Contrast enhancement is applied to captured camera images, since skin texture may not be observed due to ultrasound gels. We employ the method implemented in MATLAB, which maps the intensity values in the input image I to new values in the output image J such that 1% of data is saturated at low and high intensities of I.

4.2   Feature Point Tracking

This step is to detect feature points from the first frame, track them in the subsequent frame and then obtain the correspondence between adjacent frames. We employ the similar approach proposed by Ishii et al. [7]. Let the image frame be $f_i(n_1, n_2)$, where (n_1, n_2) is the pixel coordinate, i indicates the frame index $(0 \leq i \leq N)$ and N is the number of frames. First, feature points are detected from image $f_i(n_1, n_2)$ using the corner detection method proposed by Shi et al. [14]. We introduce parameter D to control the density of extracted feature points so as to obtain the stable localization result. If feature points are extracted from the area within $\pm D$ pixels centered on a feature point, these points are removed. Next, we find the corresponding points in subsequent image $f_{i+1}(n_1, n_2)$ from the extracted feature points in current image $f_i(n_1, n_2)$ to track the feature points. We employ a correspondence matching method using Phase-Only Correlation (POC) [18] to find accurate corresponding points. The use of POC makes it possible to obtain the translational displacement with sub-pixel accuracy between small image blocks and evaluate the similarity between images according to the correlation peak of the POC function. If the corresponding point pair has a low correlation value of the POC function, we eliminate it as an outlier. Then, we extract feature points on $f_{i+1}(n_1, n_2)$ from the area without the feature point tracked from $f_i(n_1, n_2)$. By repeating the above processes until the last frame $f_N(n_1, n_2)$, we can obtain a set of tracked feature points through a video sequence.

4.3   Structure from Motion (SfM)

This step is to estimate the rigid-body camera motion, i.e., rotation R and translation t, using SfM [4,17]. SfM repeats the linear solution and nonlinear optimization by sequentially adding images. The extrinsic camera parameters R and t of i-th image $f_i(n_1, n_2)$ are estimated in the linear solution using the method proposed by Kneip et al. [9] from the geometric relationship between the reconstructed 3D points and the coordinates of tracked feature points. Note that the extrinsic camera parameters R and t of the first two frames are estimated with the normalized five-point algorithm [11]. We also employ random sample consensus (RANSAC) [1] to robustly estimate the parameters in the first two frames. The 3D points of tracked feature points are obtained using the estimated extrinsic parameters in the i-th image $f_i(n_1, n_2)$ according to triangulation. The reconstructed 3D points and estimated camera parameters are optimized by minimizing reprojection error using bundle adjustments [4,17]. The reprojection error is defined by the Euclidean distance $||m - m_{rep}||^2$, where $m = (u, v)$ is a feature point and m_{rep} is a point obtained by projecting a 3D point $M = (X, Y, Z)$ onto the image using a projection matrix of a camera. We employ global and local bundle adjustments [17] depending on the target range in this paper. Finally, we obtain the camera motion represented by rotation R and translation t for each frame and sparse 3D point clouds. The resultant camera motion corresponds to the location of the US probe.

4.4   Coordinate Conversion

The coordinate M_c of estimated camera motion is converted into the coordinate M_p of the probe coordinate system using Eq. (5).

4.5   3D US Volume Reconstruction

This step is to reconstruct 3D US volume from a set of US images. We use Stradwin[2] to reconstruct 3D US volumes from a set of US images and their location in the 3D space obtained by the proposed method.

5   Experiments and Discussion

We evaluate the performance of the proposed method using the dataset acquired by the developed system as shown in Fig. 1. Our dataset consists of camera images and US images acquired from 2 volunteers. We scanned the area around the arm and the thigh. The travel distance of the US probe is about 200 mm for the arm and 100 mm for the thigh, respectively. The accuracy of US probe localization is evaluated by the accuracy of 3D point clouds reconstructed by SfM, since the accuracy of the camera motion is equivalent to that of 3D point clouds. A 3D mesh model of each target is measured with the laser scanner (Konica Minolta, Inc., VIVID910) for quantitative performance evaluation. The accuracy of 3D reconstruction is evaluated by comparing the reconstructed 3D point clouds and the ground-truth mesh model using the iterative closest point algorithm [19].

Figure 4 shows the ground-truth 3D model, reconstructed 3D point clouds and estimated camera position and reconstructed 3D US volume for the arm. The shape of reconstructed 3D points is almost the same as the ground-truth 3D model. We observe that the camera is moved straight from the elbow to the wrist. The Root Mean Square (RMS) of reconstruction error is about 2 mm for the probe travel distance of 200 mm. In the conventional method [16], the cumulative error of the probe localization is about 10 mm for the probe travel distance of 100 mm.

The thigh area is used to confirm the effectiveness of probe-camera calibration, since this area has the curved shape. Figure 5 shows reconstructed 3D point

---

[2] Stradwin: http://mi.eng.cam.ac.uk/~rwp/stradwin.

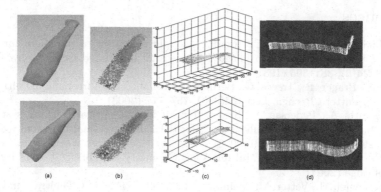

Fig. 4. Experimental results for arm area: (a) ground-truth 3D model, (b) reconstructed 3D point clouds, (c) 3D point clouds and estimated camera position and (d) reconstructed 3D US volume.

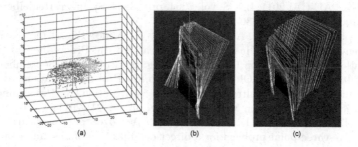

Fig. 5. Experimental results for thigh area: (a) 3D point clouds and camera position, (b) reconstructed 3D US volume without probe-camera calibration and (c) reconstructed 3D US volume with probe-camera calibration.

clouds and camera position and reconstructed 3D US volume for the thigh. The 3D US volume without probe-camera calibration is warped out of shape as shown in Fig. 5(b), while the 3D US volume with probe-camera calibration represents the curved shape of the thigh as shown in Fig. 5(c).

6   Conclusion

This paper proposed the probe-camera system for 3D US image reconstruction. This paper also proposed the simple method for probe-camera calibration and US probe localization method based on structure from motion. Through a set of experiments, we demonstrated that the location of the US probe can be estimated with about 2 mm error for the probe travel distance of 200 mm. We expect that the use of the proposed system makes it possible to enhance the effectiveness of US imaging in point-of-care, since 3D US volume can be obtained using a US probe with a camera.

References

1. Fischler, M.A., Bolles, R.C.: Random sample consensus: a paradigm for model fitting with applications to image analysis and automated cartography. Comm. ACM **24**(6), 381–395 (1981)
2. Gee, A., Prager, R., Treece, G., Berman, L.: Engineering a freehand 3D ultrasound system. Pattern Recogn. Lett. **24**(4–5), 757–777 (2003)
3. Goldsmith, A., Pedersen, P., Szabo, T.: An inertial-optical tracking system for portable, quantitative, 3D ultrasound. In: IEEE International Ultrasonics Symposium Proceedings, pp. 45–49 (2008)
4. Hartley, R., Zisserman, A.: Multiple View Geometry. Cambridge University Press, Cambridge (2004)
5. Hastenteufel, M., Vetter, M., Meinzer, H.P., Wolf, I.: Effect of 3D ultrasound probes on the accuracy of electromagnetic tracking systems. Ultrasound Med. Biol. **32**(9), 1359–1368 (2006)
6. Horvath, S., et al.: Towards an ultrasound probe with vision: structured light to determine surface orientation. In: Linte, C.A., Moore, J.T., Chen, E.C.S., Holmes, D.R. (eds.) AE-CAI 2011. LNCS, vol. 7264, pp. 58–64. Springer, Heidelberg (2012). doi:10.1007/978-3-642-32630-1_6
7. Ishii, J., Sakai, S., Ito, K., Aoki, T., Yanagi, T., Ando, T.: 3D reconstruction of urban environments using in-vehicle fisheye camera. In: Proceedings of the IEEE International Conference on Image Processing, pp. 2145–2148, September 2013
8. Ito, S., Ito, K., Aoki, T., Ohmiya, J., Kondo, S.: Probe localization using structure from motion for 3D ultrasound image reconstruction. In: Proceedings of the International Conference on Medical Imaging, pp. 68–71 (2017)
9. Kneip, L., Scaramuzza, D., Siegwart, R.: A novel parametrization of the perspective-three-point problem for a direct computation of absolute camera position and orientation. In: Proceedings of the International Conference Computer Vision and Pattern Recognition, pp. 2969–2976 (2011)
10. Lange, T., Kraft, S., Eulenstein, S., Lamecker, H., Schlag, P.: Automatic calibration of 3D ultrasound probes. In: Handels, H., Ehrhardt, J., Deserno, T., Meinzer, H.P., Tolxdorff, T. (eds.) Bildverarbeitung fur die Medizin 2011, pp. 169–173. Springer, Heidelberg (2011). doi:10.1007/978-3-642-19335-4_36
11. Nistér, D.: An efficient solution to the five-point relative pose problem. IEEE Trans. Pattern Anal. Mach. Intell. **26**(6), 756–770 (2004)
12. Rafii-Tari, H., Abolmaesumi, P., Rohling, R.: Panorama ultrasound for guiding epidural anesthesia: a feasibility study. In: Taylor, R.H., Yang, G.-Z. (eds.) IPCAI 2011. LNCS, vol. 6689, pp. 179–189. Springer, Heidelberg (2011). doi:10.1007/978-3-642-21504-9_17
13. Rousseau, F., Hellier, P., Barillot, C.: A fully automatic calibration procedure for freehand 3D ultrasound. In: Proceedings of the IEEE International Symposium Biomedical, Imaging, pp. 985–988 (2002)
14. Shi, J., Tomasi, C.: Good features to track. In: Proceedings of the International Conference on Computer Vision and Pattern Recognition, pp. 593–600 (1994)
15. Stolka, P., Kang, H., Choti, M., Boctor, E.: Multi-DoF probe trajectory reconstruction with local sensors for 2D-to-3D ultrasound. In: Proceedings of the IEEE International Symposium Biomedical, Imaging, pp. 316–319 (2010)
16. Sun, S.-Y., Gilbertson, M., Anthony, B.W.: Probe localization for freehand 3D ultrasound by tracking skin features. In: Golland, P., Hata, N., Barillot, C., Hornegger, J., Howe, R. (eds.) MICCAI 2014. LNCS, vol. 8674, pp. 365–372. Springer, Cham (2014). doi:10.1007/978-3-319-10470-6_46

17. Szeliski, R.: Computer Vision: Algorithms and Applications. Springer-Verlag New York Inc., New York (2010). doi:10.1007/978-3-642-12848-6
18. Takita, K., Muquit, M.A., Aoki, T., Higuchi, T.: A sub-pixel correspondence search for computer vision applications. IEICE Trans. Fundam. **E87−A**(8), 1913–1923 (2004)
19. Zhang, Z.: Iterative point matching for registration of free-form curves and surfaces. Int. J. Comput. Vis. **13**(2), 119–152 (1994)

Ultrasound Augmentation: Rapid 3-D Scanning for Tracking and On-Body Display

Maeliss Jallais, Hastings Greer$^{(\boxtimes)}$, Sam Gerber, Matt McCormick,
Deepak Chittajallu, Neal Siekierski, and Stephen Aylward

Kitware Inc., Carrboro, NC 27510, USA
`hastings.greer@gmail.com`

Abstract. By using a laser projector and high speed camera, we can add three capabilities to an ultrasound system: tracking the probe, tracking the patient, and projecting information onto the probe and patient. We can use these capabilities to guide an untrained operator to take high quality, well framed ultrasound images for computer-augmented, point-of-care ultrasound applications.

1 Motivation

We have developed algorithms that analyze ultrasound signals to detect internal bleeding [1] and increased intracranial pressure (increased optic nerve sheath diameter) [2]. These algorithms are part of a computer-augmented, point-of-care ultrasound (CAPCUS) system that is intended to aid in the triage of patients with abdominal or head trauma at the scene of an accident, helping emergency medical service (EMS) personnel decide when to order expedited transport and initiate life-saving measures in the field.

One of the critical, remaining challenges with deploying our CAPCUS system is informing the EMS personnel on where to place and how to manipulate an ultrasound probe at various anatomic locations in order to, for example, thoroughly examine the regions of the abdomen where blood tends to pool. This positioning task requires extensive anatomic and ultrasound training, beyond what most clinicians and/or EMS personnel typically receive.

This paper presents an innovative device that combines patient and probe tracking with augmented reality to create an "augmented ultrasound" system. It is one of a variety of methods and user interfaces that we are investigating to guide EMS personnel in probe placement, to inform them of data quality and to convey diagnoses.

2 Augmented Ultrasound

Rather than displaying data and instructions on a screen, our augmented ultrasound system proposes to concisely convey guidance and diagnoses by projecting instructions onto the surface of the patient. There are several advantages. Unlike

© Springer International Publishing AG 2017
M.J. Cardoso et al. (Eds.): BIVPCS/POCUS 2017, LNCS 10549, pp. 138–145, 2017.
DOI: 10.1007/978-3-319-67552-7_17

a screen, a projection does not require the operator to look away from the patient. In addition, when combined with a tracker, the projection can provide directions in absolute terms. For example, a CAPCUS system that uses our algorithm for on body display would be able to direct the operator to "Place the scanner on the bullseye," instead of relying on more abstract instructions such as "Place the scanner on the right side of the patient's chest, half-way between the nipple and the shoulder." Furthermore, instructions can be updated based on the tracked movement of the ultrasound probe and the images/anatomy captured in the ultrasound data, ensuring coverage of an anatomic area or flashing a warning icon when the probe is not making sufficient contact with the skin.

The augmented ultrasound system must be able to track the ultrasound probe and the surface of the patient's body and then use the generated model of the body and the position of the probe to accurately project graphics/instructions onto the patient's body. Furthermore, the augmented ultrasound system must work in sunlight and in rugged environments with minimal set-up time so that it can be applied at the scene of an accident.

In the next section, we discuss our system for forming a three-dimensional (3D) model of a scene using a laser projector and a high-speed camera. Then, we describe how we track objects in that scene.

3   3D Scene Modeling

To form a 3D model of a scene, we replicated and extended the system described in a paper by researchers at Carnegie Mellon University that performed depth from structured light reconstruction using a portable projector, which uses laser projection technology, and a high-speed camera. (See Fig. 1, adapted from [3].) The laser projector draws only one line of a projected image at a time, but it does so fast enough that the human eye only sees the complete image. The high-speed camera is capable of precise timing and fast shutter speed. These properties allow the camera to take a picture as the projector draws a specific line of the image. Through a one-time calibration of the camera and the projector, and by using structured-light reconstruction algorithms, each point on a projected line that is seen by the camera can be efficiently and accurately triangulated to a point in 3D space (i.e., each illuminated point seen in a camera image is at the intersection of the plane/line of light emitted by the projector and the corresponding pixel/line viewed by the camera). The camera/projector calibration process is adapted from the method developed at Brown University [4], which is based on OpenCV and uses the camera application programming interface (API).

Our system is composed of a Grasshopper3 camera and a SONY mobile projector MP CL1. With a resolution of 2048×1536, we can use the camera at a frame rate of 300 fps. The update rate per image of the laser projector is 60 Hz in scan line order. Given its resolution of 1920×720, it projects 43,200 lines/s.

The augmented ultrasound system works under varied lighting conditions for three reasons. First, the shutter speed simplifies the detection of which pixels are

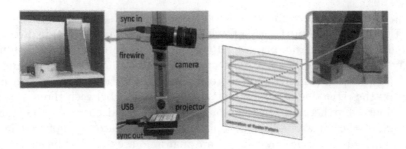

Fig. 1. The augmented reality system uses a pico projector (based on laser projection technology) to display an image in a scene. A high-speed camera sees the individual lines being drawn by the projector to create the image. Via appropriate camera calibration, custom circuitry to detect the vertical reset of the laser and depth from structured lighting algorithms, a 3D model of the scene can be formed at very high resolution in about one second. Figure adapted from [3].

Table 1. Hardware used, with prices

Device	Manufacturer	Price
Grasshopper 3 GS3-U3-32S4C-C	Point grey	$975.00
MP-CL1 Projector	Sony	$349.00
Photodiode, BPW34S	Vishay semiconductor Opto division	$6.66

illuminated by the projector. It suppresses ambient light, even direct sunlight, simply by remaining open for no more than a tiny fraction of a second (Table 1).

This benefit arises because the laser projector illuminates each point very brightly, but only for a fraction of a millisecond. Alternatively, ambient sources like the sun illuminate continuously at a lower intensity. Second, we use background subtraction to further reduce the effect of ambient light. In particular, from each image that is taken, we subtract an image from when the laser is in a different location. Third, we apply a custom method that quickly detects the brightest point on a vertical scan line in a grayscale image.

The most difficult challenge with our low-cost, compact ultrasound augmentation system was that the horizontal sync signal produced by the projector/HDMI protocol was not phase-locked to the actual vertical movement of the laser. For this reason, we opted to trigger the camera off the light emitted by the projector, using a photocell and a pair of Operational Amplifiers. This horizontal sync is critically important because it is needed to determine which line is being projected at any point in time. The amplifier circuit converts the noisy photocell into a digital trigger signal. See Fig. 2.

Example reconstructions generated by the system are shown in Fig. 3.

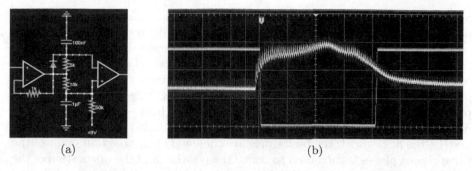

Fig. 2. (a) Circuit diagram of the photo detector system used to determine when the laser returns to the upper left and begins drawing a new image (approximately every 1/60th of a second). (b) Oscilloscope-measured photocell output (yellow) and circuit output (blue) signals. The circuit output's falling edge is used as a camera trigger. (Color figure online)

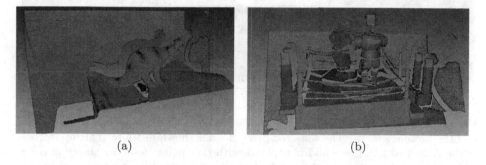

(a)   (b)

Fig. 3. Examples of 3D scenes captured by our system.

4   Object Tracking

Having formed a 3D model of a scene, the next step in ultrasound augmentation is to track an ultrasound probe. To that end, we mounted a multi-cubed, color-tagged marker (designed by InnerOptic) on the probe. The colors of the cube are red, blue and green. They are optimized for the response curves of the color detectors in the camera. By determining the intersection of three adjacent faces on the cubes, we can determine the position and the orientation of the ultrasound probe.

To simplify and speed the tracking algorithm, instead of estimating the specific location of each cube face, we estimate the planes that contain each of the faces of the cube and then solve for the intersection of those planes. The plane detection method begins with color pixel detection, using statistical models of the appearance of the cube faces under a range of lighting conditions. Depending on the image from the projector, the ambient light and the adjacent objects in the environment, extraneous pixels may be incorrectly identified as cube pixels based on color alone. To eliminate extraneous pixels, we compute the centers of gravity for each target color using robust statistics. Knowing the expected position of each face relative to the others, we can redefine the estimates of the centers of gravity by eliminating colored pixels that are inconsistent with the centers of gravity or with the expected relative positions of each face. To further reduce the influence of extraneous pixels, we also estimate the equations of the planes using the random sample consensus (RANSAC) algorithm. It randomly picks three points, computes the plane defined by them and then scores that plane based on how many other cube points are included in that plane. Ultimately, the planes with the best scores are chosen. The intersection point of the three chosen planes is then used to define the position and the orientation of the probe in space. A sample result of three detected planes intersecting the scene is shown in Fig. 4.

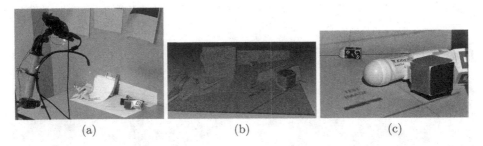

(a)   (b)   (c)

Fig. 4. (a) The setup of the system, with the projector at the top left and the camera and the bottom left. (b) The collected point cloud is shown in white. The intersection of the estimated red, green and blue planes with that point cloud are shown in color. This indicates that the faces of the cube are well represented by the estimated planes. (c) A close-up of the scene shows the projected colored planes and a projected yellow instruction card (labeled "test image") that automatically follows the tip of the ultrasound probe. (Color figure online)

Our camera is capable of up to 300 frames per second, and our projector runs at 60 sweeps per second. However, running the camera at full frame rate does not result in an even coverage of the scene by the captured images. In addition, some frames are not useful because they would be captured as the laser is returning to the top of the screen. Finally, it is only possible to trigger the camera at evenly spaced intervals, a variable delay after our optical detection circuit fires. In our system, the camera fires three times every time the optical detection circuit is activated by the laser, leading to a speed of 180 lines per second, which is equivalent to 4 reconstructions per second.

Our system can trade frame rate for resolution of the point cloud, so we tested the precision of tracking for a variety of point cloud resolutions. The results of this test are shown in Fig. 5. We found that precision did not improve past 45 lines per frame, achieving a standard deviation of 1.2 mm per axis. We also investigated the shape of this error, finding it to be roughly isotropic, as shown if Fig. 6.

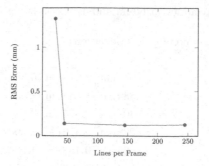

Fig. 5. The behavior of error as the number of lines per reconstruction is increased at a distance of 60 cm

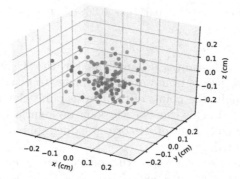

Fig. 6. Representative error in x, y, and z at a distance of 60 cm with 45 lines per reconstruction

5   Projecting onto the Scene

Once the complete system has captured a point cloud, located the ultrasound probe, and determined a diagnosis from the ultrasound data, the system must display the results onto the patient's skin. The position of the displayed results should be relative to the probe and undistorted, i.e., "rectified" with respect to the surface onto which they are being projected. To aid in this goal, display elements, such as text annotations, images, and arrows, are specified in 3-D world coordinates. We support commands such as "Color yellow all points within a 4 cm radius of the world-point $(60, -12, 3)$" or "Project the text 'Poor Contact: Apply pressure' at the point 5 cm in front of the ultrasound probe."

To achieve this effect, we use a stored, high resolution point cloud known as the "canvas" that is captured during initialization and updated only when the rapidly acquired reconstructions begin to deviate from the canvas. The canvas point cloud has up to 700 lines, whereas rapid point clouds used for tracking have only 45 lines.

Graphics primitives such as spheres or images as well as ray tracings and volume renderings are drawn onto the canvas, by updating the color associated

Table 2. Accuracy at 60 cm and 400 lx on 300 acquisitions

Lines on cube	Std deviation		
	x	y	z
4	3.001 cm	2.248 cm	6.846 cm
5	0.884 cm	1.134 cm	2.937 cm
6	0.301 cm	0.875 cm	3.075 cm
7	0.229 cm	0.570 cm	1.000 cm
8	0.105 cm	0.455 cm	1.234 cm
10	0.074 cm	0.087 cm	0.084 cm
20	0.065 cm	0.077 cm	0.062 cm
30	0.057 cm	0.070 cm	0.062 cm
40	0.057 cm	0.068 cm	0.055 cm

with each point. Next, the canvas is transformed by the "Camera Matrix" of the projector, which takes points from world coordinates to pixel coordinates on the projected image. Finally, the points of the canvas point cloud are splatted onto a bitmap and projected. This causes each point on a surface in the scene to be illuminated with the color light of its corresponding approximate nearest point in the canvas pointcloud.

The four frames per second reconstruction rate may seem slow, but our system does not need to rely on a high frame rate to avoid nausea or support smooth navigation. Only the annotations, not the full scene, are being driven by the system. Additionally, the ultrasound probe is typically a slow moving object and the environment is generally relatively static. See Table 2.

6   Conclusion

Ongoing work focuses on quantifying the performance of this algorithm. Experiments presented in this paper indicate 2 mm consistency within a 30 cm × 60 cm × 60 cm operating environment, updated at four frames per second. In other experiments, not presented in this paper, the system has been shown to be insensitive to a wide range of ambient light brightness and to the image being projected into the scene.

In future work, the probe tracker data will be used, in combination with a custom image reconstruction technique, to compound a sequence of imprecisely and sparsely tracked ultrasound images into a complete 3D Volume. In that volume, vessels, for example, could be identified and the scene could be augmented with instructions on where to insert the needle, at what angle, and to what depth, so as to best intersect with a target vessel. This is illustrated in Fig. 7.

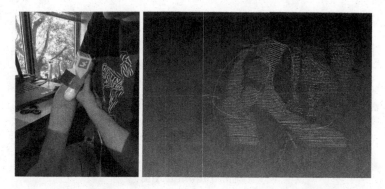

Fig. 7. An illustration of the end goal of the system. A target (black X) is projected onto the skin as the camera computes depth from structured light using the raster lines of the projected image as that image is drawn. Ultrasound can be used to detect peripheral vessels, select needle insertion locations and verify needle placement patency.

Acknowledgments. This work was funded, in part, by the following grants.
- NIH/NIBIB: In-field FAST procedure support and automation (R43EB016621)
- NIH/NINDS: Multimodality image-based assessment system for traumatic brain injury (R44NS081792)
- NIH/NIGMS/NIBIB: Slicer+PLUS: Collaborative, open-source software for ultrasound analysis (R01EB021396)

References

1. Aylward, S.R., McCormick, M., Kang, H.J., Razzaque, S., Kwitt, R., Niethammer, M.: Ultrasound spectroscopy. In: 2016 IEEE 13th International Symposium on Biomedical Imaging (ISBI), pp. 1013–1016. IEEE (2016)
2. Gerber, S., Jallais, M., Greer, H., McCormick, M., Montgomery, S., Freeman, B., Kane, D., Chittajallu, D., Siekierski, N., Aylward, S.: Automatic estimation of the optic nerve sheath diameter from ultrasound images. In: MICCAI Workshop (2017)
3. Mertz, C., Koppal, S.J., Sia, S., Narasimhan, S.: A low-power structured light sensor for outdoor scene reconstruction and dominant material identification. In: 2012 IEEE Computer Society Conference on Computer Vision and Pattern Recognition Workshops (CVPRW), pp. 15–22. IEEE (2012)
4. Moreno, D., Taubin, G.: Simple, accurate, and robust projector-camera calibration. In: 2012 Second International Conference on 3D Imaging, Modeling, Processing, Visualization and Transmission (3DIMPVT), pp. 464–471. IEEE (2012)

Overall Proficiency Assessment in Point-of-Care Ultrasound Interventions: The Stopwatch is not Enough

Matthew S. Holden[✉], Zsuzsanna Keri, Tamas Ungi,
and Gabor Fichtinger

School of Computing, Queen's University, Kingston, Canada
72mh@queensu.ca

Abstract. With the shift in the medical education curriculum to a competency-based model, objective proficiency assessment is necessary. In this work, we use exploratory factor analysis to assess which primitive metrics convey unique information about proficiency in point-of-care ultrasound applications. We retrospectively validate the proposed methods on three datasets: FAST examination, femoral line, and lumbar puncture. We identify a minimal set of metrics for proficiency assessment in each application. Furthermore, we validate that overall proficiency assessment methods are unaffected by the removal of redundant metrics. This work demonstrates that proficiency in point-of-care ultrasound applications is multi-faceted, and that measuring completion time alone is not enough and application-specific metrics have added value in proficiency assessment.

Keywords: Surgical skills assessment · Ultrasound-guided interventions

1   Introduction

Medical education is undergoing a shift from a traditional time-based model to a competency based model, where trainees graduate only upon achieving a competency benchmark. With increasing demands on expert clinician time, this necessitates automatic methods for proficiency assessment.

Accordingly, there has been a proliferation of methods of objective, automatic technical proficiency assessment for many clinical applications. These methods perform computation on data from a different sources including: hand or tool motion tracking data, video data of the surgical field or operating room, surgeon status information from wearable sensors (e.g. eye gaze, cognitive load, muscle activity), or quantification of resulting tissue. Reviews of methods for proficiency assessment for medical interventions training can be found in [1, 2].

Computing overall proficiency from a combination of primitive performance metrics is common practice. This is because primitive metrics are straightforward to compute, easy for trainees to understand, and readily interpreted into actionable feedback. Furthermore, they can be used to capture application-specific information that generic assessment methods cannot. Fraser et al. and Stylopoulos et al. first

© Springer International Publishing AG 2017
M.J. Cardoso et al. (Eds.): BIVPCS/POCUS 2017, LNCS 10549, pp. 146–153, 2017.
DOI: 10.1007/978-3-319-67552-7_18

addressed this, proposing a sum of normalized features [3] and a sum of z-scores [4], respectively. Subsequently, Allen et al. showed that using support vector machines for overall proficiency classification outperformed either of these methods [5]. Oropesa et al. confirmed that support vector machines likewise outperform linear discriminant analysis and adaptive-neuro fuzzy inference for classification overall proficiency classification [6]. Modern machine learning techniques have also been applied to this problem [7].

It is interesting to consider which metrics are critical for overall proficiency assessment and which metrics are redundant. Primarily, metrics must be valid for distinguishing novices from experts. Several valid metrics used in the assessment, however, may measure the same aspect of proficiency and correlate strongly, while others may address different aspects of proficiency. Redundant metrics may be removed to reduce system complexity without reducing assessment accuracy or feedback quality. Metrics addressing different aspects of proficiency, on the other hand, must remain to achieve a complete assessment with feedback specific to each aspect of proficiency.

In this work, we seek to evaluate which primitive metrics are sufficient and necessary for a complete assessment of technical proficiency in point-of-care ultrasound applications. In particular, we address whether simply measuring completion time is sufficient for overall proficiency assessment and the role of application-specific metrics.

2 Methods

2.1 Primitive Metric Validity

While most primitive metrics are designed to measure a clinically important quantity, it must still be show that they correlate with proficiency. To this end, we examined primitive metrics from both novices and experts, and assessed whether there is a difference between metrics for the two groups. Metrics which did not show evidence of validity were removed from subsequent analysis.

First, we used the Mann-Whitney U test ($\alpha = 0.05$) to determine if there is a statistically significant difference between the two groups for each metric. We used Cliff's Δ to quantify the effect size. Additionally, we measured the information gain associated with splitting on each metric. The information gain indicates how well splitting the data improves the groups' purity, where large information gain indicates that a metric distinguishes novices from experts effectively. We further assessed if the split produced significantly different groups using Fisher's exact test ($\alpha = 0.05$).

2.2 Primitive Metric Redundancy

Metric redundancy is most commonly computed using correlation, where a strong correlation indicates a high likelihood of redundancy. As an initial check, we computed the correlation between each pair of metrics.

Subsequently, we performed Exploratory Factor Analysis (EFA) on the primitive metric values. EFA expresses each primitive metric as a linear combination of some set of latent factors. Two primitive metrics which are similar linear combinations of the latent factors would be considered redundant. Furthermore, when combined with expert knowledge, the latent factors can be interpreted as aspects of technical proficiency and their importance can be identified. For this study, we used the principal components methods and chose the smallest number of factors explaining at least 90% of the variance in the data. Two primitive metrics were considered redundant if they both had loading factors greater than 0.90 on the same latent factor.

2.3   Assessment Using Non-redundant Primitive Metrics

Once we identified which metrics were redundant using EFA, for each set of redundant metrics we chose one "representative" metric. This metric was chosen to be the metric with the best loading on each of the latent factors. We then computed an overall proficiency classification for each participant using the "representative" metrics for both the traditional sum of z-scores method [4] and the support vector machine method [5]. For the sum of z-scores method we used equal weighting. For the support vector machine method, we normalized the data on the range [0, 1] and used the radial basis function.

We compared the proficiency classification accuracies achieved using the "representative" set of primitive metrics with the accuracies achieved using all primitive metrics. The area under the receiver-operator characteristics curves was computed for each metric set for each of the sum of z-scores method and the support vector machine method. We determined whether the areas under the curves was different for the metric sets using the Hanley-McNeil test ($\alpha = 0.05$).

2.4   Datasets

We retrospectively analyzed datasets from three point-of-care ultrasound training applications: FAST ultrasound examination, femoral line insertion, and freehand lumbar puncture. In each case, we used previously computed metric values based on tool tracking data. In each case, the metrics were specifically designed by experts to capture relevant information on proficiency while performing the intervention.

In the FAST ultrasound training dataset, a group of fourteen novices and fifteen intermediates performed a complete FAST examination on a healthy volunteer on each of the four regions of interest (hepatorenal, splenorenal, pericardial, and pelvic regions) [8]. The ultrasound probe was tracked relative to the volunteer, and the following primitive metrics were computed: completion time, percentage of expert-defined points of interest missed, and ultrasound probe path length.

The femoral line insertion dataset included ten novices and four experts performing an ultrasound-guided insertion on a commercially available simulation phantom [9]. The motion of the operators' hands was tracked relative to the phantom model, and the following primitive metrics were computed: completion time, probe hand path length, needle hand path length, probe hand rotational actions, needle hand rotational actions, probe hand translational actions, and needle hand translational actions.

The lumbar puncture dataset included twenty-three novices and five experts performing freehand lumbar puncture on a commercially available lumbar spine model [10].

The pose of the operators' hands and needle was tracked relative to the phantom model, and the following primitive metrics were computed: completion time, left hand path length, right hand path length, needle tip path length, tissue damage caused by needle, needle tip path length in tissue, and needle tip time in tissue.

3   Results

3.1   Primitive Metric Validity

For the FAST dataset, all metrics were significantly different between novices and intermediates, thus all metrics were kept for subsequent analysis. For the femoral line dataset, probe hand and needle hand rotational actions were not significantly different between novices and experts, thus these two metrics were removed. All other femoral line metrics were kept. For the lumbar puncture dataset, all metrics were significantly different between the novice and expert groups, thus all metrics were kept (Table 1).

Table 1. Validity of metrics for each dataset. MW indicates the p-value for the Mann-Whitney test; Δ indicates the non-parametric effect size; F indicates the p-value for Fisher's exact test; IG indicates the maximal information gain associated with splitting on that metric.

Dataset	Metric	MW	Δ	F	IG
FAST	Completion time (s)	<0.001	0.40	<0.001	0.10
	Points missed (%)	<0.001	0.58	<0.001	0.21
	Probe path length (mm)	<0.001	0.44	<0.001	0.08
Femoral Line	Completion time (s)	0.002	1.00	<0.001	0.60
	Probe hand path length (mm)	0.024	0.80	0.015	0.33
	Needle hand path length (mm)	0.024	0.80	0.011	0.36
	Probe hand rotational actions	0.056	0.68	0.070	0.26
	Needle hand rotational actions	0.607	0.20	0.221	0.16
	Probe hand translational actions	0.006	0.93	0.005	0.42
	Needle hand translational actions	0.002	1.00	<0.001	0.60
Lumbar Puncture	Completion time (s)	<0.001	1.00	<0.001	0.47
	Left hand path length (mm)	0.001	0.93	<0.001	0.32
	Right hand path length (mm)	0.007	0.79	0.003	0.22
	Needle tip path length (mm)	0.006	0.81	0.001	0.23
	Tissue damage (mm^2)	0.010	0.76	0.001	0.25
	Needle path in tissue (mm)	0.026	0.65	0.026	0.14
	Needle time in tissue (s)	0.022	0.67	0.008	0.15

3.2   Primitive Metric Redundancy

The correlation matrices for each dataset are shown in Fig. 1. Using EFA, two latent factors were found for the FAST dataset, accounting for 91% of the variance. Two latent factors were found for the femoral line dataset, accounting for 98% of the variance. Three latent factors were found for the lumbar puncture dataset, accounting for 93% of the variance. The loading plots for each dataset are present in Fig. 2.

For the FAST dataset, completion time and probe path length both primarily load on one latent factor, and points missed loads primarily on the other latent factor. We interpret the first latent factor to be "efficiency" and the second latent factor to be "thoroughness". For the femoral line dataset, needle hand path length loads primarily on one latent factor and probe hand translational actions loads primarily on the other latent factor. We conjecture the first latent factor to be "needle hand efficiency" and the second latent factor to be "probe hand efficiency". All other primitive metrics cross-load on the two latent factors. For the lumbar puncture dataset, tissue damage caused by needle, needle tip path length in tissue, and time needle in tissue load primarily on one factor, left hand path length and right hand path length load primarily on another, and needle tip path length loads primarily on a third factor. Completion time cross-loads. We hypothesize these three latent factors to be respectively "needle insertion efficiency", "landmarking efficiency", and "needle placement efficiency".

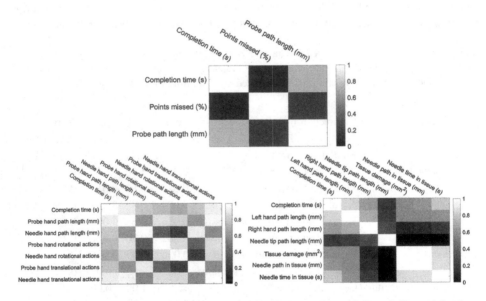

Fig. 1. Correlation matrices for metrics in the FAST (top), femoral line (left), and lumbar puncture (right) datasets. White indicates high correlation; black indicates low correlation.

Based on the primitive metric loadings, the following metrics were kept as "representative" metrics. For the FAST dataset, completion time and points missed were kept. For the femoral line dataset, needle hand path length and probe hand translational actions were kept. For the lumbar puncture dataset, right hand path length, needle tip path length, and tissue damage were kept.

3.3   Assessment Using Non-redundant Primitive Metrics

Differences in the areas under the curves using all primitive metrics and using a "representative" set were insignificant for all datasets using both the sum of z-scores

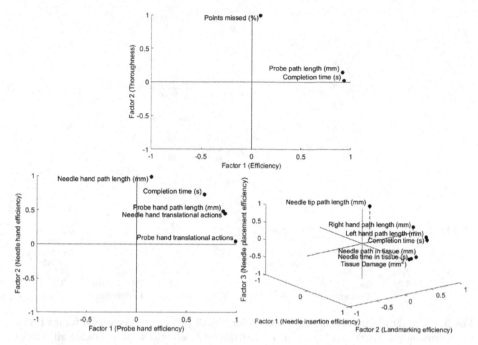

Fig. 2. Loading plots for metrics onto presumed factors in the FAST (top), femoral line (left), and lumbar puncture (right) datasets.

Table 2. Area under the curve (AUC) for each method of overall proficiency assessment. All AUC indicates the area under the curve using all metrics, and Rep. AUC indicates the area under the curve using only the "representative metrics". p-value indicates the p-value for the Hanley-McNeil test.

Dataset	Sum of Z-Scores			Support Vector Machine		
	All AUC	Rep. AUC	p-value	All AUC	Rep. AUC	p-value
FAST	0.84	0.83	0.45	0.84	0.84	0.44
Femoral line	1.00	1.00	0.50	1.00	1.00	0.50
Lumbar puncture	0.97	0.91	0.31	1.00	0.96	0.25

and support vector machine methods (Table 2). The greatest change in area under the curve was 0.052, for the lumbar puncture dataset using the z-score method (Fig. 3).

4   Discussion and Conclusion

In each dataset, the majority of the reported metrics were determined to be valid. There were strong correlations between many of the metrics, and exploratory factor analysis indicated that the metrics were associated with two to three latent factors. We interpreted

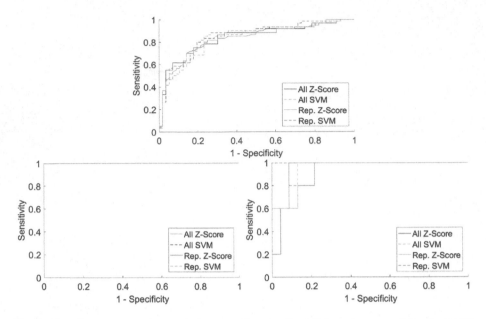

Fig. 3. Receiver operator characteristic curves for overall proficiency assessment for the FAST (top), femoral line (left), and lumbar puncture (right) datasets. Black lines indicate all metrics were used; red lines indicate only "representative" metrics were used. Solid lines indicate the sum of z-scores method was used; dashed lines indicate the support vector machine method was used. (Color figure online)

the meaning of these latent factors using domain-specific knowledge. Taking only the most representative metrics for each factor, we achieved accuracies for overall proficiency assessment that were not significantly different from accuracies using all metrics. This indicates that many of the metrics could be removed; however, completion time cannot be used alone to measure proficiency. Furthermore, it shows application-specific primitive metrics have added value in proficiency assessment.

This study, however, is not without limitations. Primarily, for the femoral line and lumbar puncture datasets, the sample size is limited with the expert group including four and five participants respectively. This can be especially problematic for EFA. The other main limitation is that we have used experience as a proxy for ground-truth proficiency. This does not account for experts who have developed bad habits or have an "off day". Ideally, ground-truth proficiency should be determined by a panel of experts using a valid objective assessment tool. Finally, our analysis assumes a monotonic relation between each metric and proficiency, which may not always be the case.

We suggest that these results will extend to other ultrasound-guided and freehand interventions. Here we have tested three different interventions, and our metric reduction techniques seem to apply well to each application, yielding less than six percent difference in proficiency classification for all datasets. We suggest this analysis could be used in other point-of-care ultrasound applications to identify which primitive metrics may be removed to reduce setup complexity and factors contributing to proficiency.

Finally, for each of these datasets, we have more than one latent factor contributing to proficiency. In particular, the application-specific metrics have added value and completion time alone is insufficient for assessing these factors. In fact, there may be additional factors which are not measured by the primitive metrics we chose. One should be aware of all such factors when computing an overall proficiency score. We suggest that providing a report card that addresses each of these factors may better allow trainees to understand which aspects of their intervention require the most improvement.

References

1. Reiley, C.E., Lin, H.C., Yuh, D.D., Hager, G.D.: Review of methods for objective surgical skill evaluation. Surg. Endosc. **25**(2), 356–366 (2011)
2. Vedula, S.S., Ishii, M., Hager, G.D.: Objective assessment of surgical technical skill and competency in the operating room. Annu. Rev. Biomed. Eng. **19**(1), 301–325 (2017)
3. Fraser, S.A., Klassen, D.R., Feldman, L.S., Ghitulescu, G.A., Stanbridge, D., Fried, G.M.: Evaluating laparoscopic skills. Surg. Endosc. Other Interv. Tech. **17**(6), 964–967 (2003)
4. Stylopoulos, N., et al.: Computer-enhanced laparoscopic training system (CELTS): bridging the gap. Surg. Endosc. **18**(5), 782–789 (2004)
5. Allen, B., Nistor, V., Dutson, E., Carman, G., Lewis, C., Faloutsos, P.: Support vector machines improve the accuracy of evaluation for the performance of laparoscopic training tasks. Surg. Endosc. **24**(1), 170–178 (2010)
6. Oropesa, I., et al.: Supervised classification of psychomotor competence in minimally invasive surgery based on instruments motion analysis. Surg. Endosc. **28**(2), 657–670 (2014)
7. Kramer, B.D., Losey, D.P., O'Malley, M.K.: SOM and LVQ classification of endovascular surgeons using motion-based metrics. In: Merényi, E., Mendenhall, M.J., O'Driscoll, P. (eds.) Advances in Self-Organizing Maps and Learning Vector Quantization. AISC, vol. 428, pp. 227–237. Springer, Cham (2016). doi:10.1007/978_3_319_28518_1_20
8. Holden, M.S., Ungi, T., McKaigney, C., Bell, C., Rang, L., Fichtinger, G.: Objective evaluation of sonographic skill in focussed assessment with sonography for trauma examinations. In: CARS 2015—Computer Assisted Radiology and Surgery Proceedings of the 29th International Congress and Exhibition Barcelona, pp. S79–S80 (2015)
9. McGraw, R., et al.: Development and evaluation of a simulation-based curriculum for ultrasound-guided central venous catheterization. CJEM **18**, 1–9 (2016)
10. Yeo, C.T., Davison, C., Ungi, T., Holden, M., Fichtinger, G., McGraw, R.: Examination of learning trajectories for simulated lumbar puncture training using hand motion analysis. Acad. Emerg. Med. **22**(10), 1187–1195 (2015)

A Novel Ultrasound Imaging Method for 2D Temperature Monitoring of Thermal Ablation

Chloé Audigier[1,2](✉), Younsu Kim[1], and Emad Boctor[1,2]

[1] Department of Computer Science, Johns Hopkins University, Baltimore, MD, USA
caudigi1@jhmi.edu
[2] Department of Radiology, Johns Hopkins University, Baltimore, MD, USA

Abstract. Accurate temperature monitoring is a crucial task that directly affects the safety and effectiveness of thermal ablation procedures.

Compared to MRI, ultrasound-based temperature monitoring systems have many advantages, including higher temporal resolution, low cost, safety, mobility and ease of use. However, conventional ultrasound (US) images have a limited accuracy due to a weak temperature sensitivity. As a result, it is more challenging to fully meet the clinical requirements for assessing the completion of ablation therapy.

A novel imaging method for temperature monitoring is proposed based on the injection of virtual US pattern in the US brightness mode (B-mode) image coupled with biophysical simulation of heat propagation. This proposed imaging method does not require any hardware extensions to the conventional US B-mode system. The main principle is to establish a bi-directional US communication between the US imaging machine and an active element inserted within the tissue. A virtual pattern can then directly be created into the US B-mode display during the ablation by controlling the timing and amplitude of the US field generated by the active element. Changes of the injected pattern are related to the change of the ablated tissue temperature through the additional knowledge of a biophysical model of heat propagation in the tissue. Those changes are monitored during ablation, generating accurate spatial and temporal temperature maps.

We demonstrated *in silico* the method feasibility and showed experimentally its applicability on a clinical US scanner using *ex vivo* data. Promising results are achieved: a mean temperature error smaller than 4 °C was achieved in all the simulation experiments. The system performance is tested under different configurations of noise in the data. The effect of error in the localization of the RFA probe is also evaluated.

1 Introduction

The use of image-guided thermal therapy has considerably expanded in the past decades. But a major limitation is still the lack of detailed thermal information

The original version of this chapter was revised: An acknowledgment has been added. The erratum to this chapter is available at https://doi.org/10.1007/978-3-319-67552-7_20

M.J. Cardoso et al. (Eds.): BIVPCS/POCUS 2017, LNCS 10549, pp. 154–162, 2017.
DOI: 10.1007/978-3-319-67552-7_19

available. Temperatures are routinely measured invasively with thermocouples, providing only sparse measurements at some single local points, resulting in less information than it might be necessary to produce satisfactory temperature distributions for assessing properly the delivered thermal dose. Several medical imaging modalities have been proposed, tested, and employed like MRI [2], which is used routinely to guide high intensity focused ultrasound (HIFU) in clinical settings to treat uterine fibroids [9]. Nevertheless, compared to MRI, ultrasound-based temperature monitoring remains particularly attractive in simplicity, mobility, accessibility, and cost. It can also provide thermal images with higher temporal and spatial resolutions.

Different methods have been proposed to use ultrasound (US) for temperature monitoring. They exploit either echo shifts due to changes in tissue thermal expansion, attenuation coefficient, speed of sound (SoS), or frequency variations, nonlinearity parameters, elasticity, or change in the backscattered energy from tissue inhomogeneities [5]. But those existing temperature monitoring methods have not yet provided a solution that effectively solves the problem of covering the entire range of temperature reached during ablation. The relationship between SoS and temperature is parabolic; therefore, the correspondence between echo-strain and temperature is not unique. Those methods also suffer from low SNR and uncertainties in the US speckles. Moreover, they rely on a reference usually measured before ablation, which makes them subject to motion artefacts.

In this work, we propose a new imaging method for temperature monitoring based on the injection of virtual pattern with high SNR in the US brightness mode (B-mode) image [3], whose deformations are easily tracked. This novel imaging method does not require any hardware extensions to the conventional US B-mode system. As the SoS and attenuation coefficient change during the ablation with the change in temperature, we show that the US information provided by the virtual injected pattern combined with a biophysical model-based simulation can be reconstructed into tomographic temperature maps. This method has the potential to monitor temperature in a two dimensional (2D) image during ablation without the need of costly MRI. Although the proposed US monitoring method could be applied to all thermal therapies based on tissue heat absorption (e.g. laser, radiofrequency (RFA), microwave, HIFU), this paper focuses on RFA. In this contribution, we first introduce the proposed method. Then, we present simulation experiments to validate its feasibility and a preliminary design for *ex vivo* implementation.

2   Methods

The different steps of the method are illustrated in Fig. 1. US B-mode images with pattern injection (PI) are simulated with their corresponding thermal maps using a biophysical thermal ablation model to constitute a simulation-based learning tool. As a new B-mode with PI is acquired during ablation, it is evaluated with the learning tool to recover the corresponding thermal map.

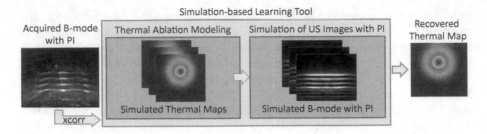

Fig. 1. Main steps of the proposed method. *See text for details.*

2.1 Active Ultrasound Pattern Injection (PI)

The proposed method requires the insertion in the targeted tissue of an active element, made of a 2 mm diameter tube shape Lead Zirconate Titate material: PZT-5H. With some hardware adjustment, it could be attached to the RFA probe, which will not increase the procedure invasiveness. A MCU-based control system is built to establish a bi-directional ultrasound (US) communication between this active element and a US machine. The active element transmits US pulses at the designated timing after line and trigger signals from the US machine are detected [4], creating a virtual pattern injection (PI) onto the original B-mode images. As the active US pulse travels back to the imaging probe, it appears as a bright spot on the B-mode image at a given location depending on the timing, frequency, duration and amplitude of the active echo pulses. Any virtual pattern can be injected onto the B-mode image, without the need of any hardware or software modification to the US machine.

2.2 Simulation-Based Learning Tool

The temperature is estimated based on two physical phenomena: the speed of sound (SoS) and attenuation thermal dependencies. The former is described as a third order polynomial [7]. In most tissue media except fatty tissues, SoS increases with temperature before reaching a plateau around 60 °C (Fig. 2, left). The latter is described by a second order polynomial derived from measurements [8] in a wide range of temperatures (Fig. 2, right). The local temperature-induced changes of SoS and attenuation in the tissue during ablation modify the virtual PI. These modifications are observed on the acquired B-mode image and can be related to temperature changes in the ablated tissue. As a new B-mode image is acquired with modification in the virtual PI, it is evaluated with the simulation-based learning tool using normalized 2D cross-correlation to recover the corresponding thermal map. In this work, the simulation-based learning tool is made of two parts described in the following sections.

Thermal Ablation Modeling. The thermal diffusion in the tissue surrounding the RFA probe can be described by the bioheat equation, as proposed in

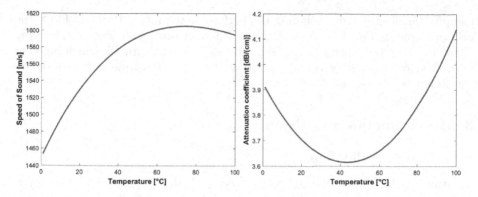

Fig. 2. Speed of sound and attenuation coefficient as functions of temperature.

the Pennes model [6]. The temperature T is modeled by solving the following reaction-diffusion equation:

$$\rho_t c_t \frac{\partial T}{\partial t} = Q + \nabla \cdot (d_t T) + R(T_{b0} - T) \tag{1}$$

where ρ_t, c_t, d_t are the density, heat capacity, conductivity of the tissue and Q is the source term. T_{b0} is the blood temperature and R is the reaction coefficient that models the blood perfusion. R is set to zero as *ex vivo* data are considered in this study. Equation 1 is solved using the Lattice Boltzmann Method (LBM) [1] implemented on general purpose Graphics Processing Units (GPU) for fast computation. A Multiple-Relaxation-Time (MRT) model on an isotropic Cartesian grid with 7-connectivity topology is used, and Neumann boundary conditions at the boundaries of the considered domain are employed. The computations are done with a time step of $\delta t = 0.01\,\text{s}$ and a spatial resolution of $\delta x = 1\,\text{mm}$, with parameters values from [1]. A realistic heating profile is imposed at the probe tip as a Dirichlet boundary condition. This model generates longitudinal 3D temperature maps, which are then converted into SoS and attenuation maps using the relationships from Fig. 2.

Simulation of US Images with PI. At any given ablation time point, a US B-mode image with temperature-induced changes in the virtual pattern is simulated based on the heterogeneous SoS and attenuation maps derived from the thermal ablation model presented above.

The nonlinear US propagation in heterogeneous medium is simulated using a nonlinear k-space model [10]. To mimic the *ex vivo* experiment protocol, a linear probe of 128 rectangular transducer elements is simulated using the k-Wave MATLAB toolbox[1]. Four active source lines around 4 mm apart from each others and driven by a four cycle tone burst with a center frequency of 1.5 MHz are simulated to model the virtual pattern injected in the *ex vivo* experiments. The

---

[1] http://www.k-wave.org.

computational grid used including the perfect match layer (PML) is 148 × 106 grid points with a grid point spacing of 4.7 mm. A delay and sum beamforming algorithm is used to reconstruct the US B-mode images with PI, which together with their corresponding thermal maps at each ablation time point constitute the simulation-based learning tool.

3   Experiments and Results

3.1   *In silico* Validation

To study its feasibility, the method is first evaluated *in silico*. We used thermal maps derived from the RFA simulation as ground truth to simulate the acquisition of B-mode images with PI every 1 s. To recover the corresponding thermal map, we chose the ablation time maximizing the maximum value of the normalized 2D cross-correlation between the considered B-mode image with PI and each of the simulated B-mode images of the simulation-based learning tool. In this case, we manage to recover the accurate thermal map in 5 s without any error as expected since the learning tool was created in a similar manner.

3.2   Sensitivity Analysis

Effect of Signal Noise. To emulate a more realistic clinical environment, the effect of noise in the amplitude of the acquired data is studied. Different Gaussian noise realizations are added to the simulated channel data with a Signal to Noise Ratio (SNR) ranging from 10 to 1. At each ablation time point, the proposed method is used to recover the actual ablation time (Fig. 3, left) and thus also the temperature map from the simulation-based learning tool. (Fig. 3, right) shows that the smaller the SNR is, the larger the error is. In the red circle, some outlier points are observed at around 600 s. At this time, the RFA stops and a cooling period starts, resulting in a small error in the recovered ablation time that can

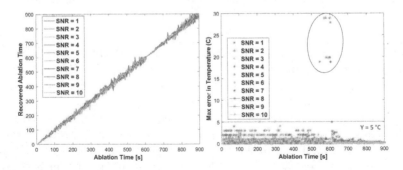

Fig. 3. (Left) Time of the recovered thermal map over the ablation time. (Right) Max error in temperature between the recovered thermal map and the ground truth for Gaussian noise configurations with different SNR.

Table 1. Time average and maximum of the max error in the 2D images for Gaussian noise configurations with different SNR.

	mean (°C)	max (°C)
SNR = 1	1.2	28.8
SNR = 2	1.3	28.8
SNR = 3	0.9	19.8
SNR = 4	0.7	18.8
SNR = 5	1.1	19.8
SNR = 6	0.5	3.0
SNR = 7	0.7	19.8
SNR = 8	0.4	2.0
SNR = 9	0.4	3.0
SNR = 10	0.4	2.0

give a large maximal error in temperature. However, one observes that most of the maximal errors are below 5 °C. Quantitative time average and maximal errors for the different Gaussian noise realizations are reported in Table 1. With a mean error of 1.2 °C in the recovered thermal map for SNR = 1, the proposed method is robust to the presence of noise in the amplitude of the signal data.

Effect of RFA Probe Mislocalization. Knowing the actual position of the ablation probe is paramount to simulate the virtual PI and thus to generate the simulation-based learning tool. This position can be determined by a preoperative US image, but could be affected by localization errors. To study this effect, a shift of 1 mm to 7 mm in the RFA probe position is introduced when simulating the acquisition of a new B-mode image, resulting in different SoS and

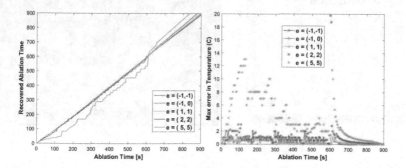

Fig. 4. (Left) Time of the recovered thermal map over the ablation time. (Right) Max error in temperature between the recovered thermal map and the ground truth for different displacements **e** (in mm) of the RFA probe position.

Table 2. Time average and maximum of the max error in the 2D images for different displacements e (in mm) of the RFA probe position.

	mean (°C)	max (°C)
e = (-1,-1)	0.6	2.0
e = (-1, 0)	0.5	2.0
e = (1, 1)	0.3	2.0
e = (2, 2)	1.0	19.7
e = (5, 5)	4.0	13.0

attenuation maps and thus a modified B-mode image. As illustrated in Fig. 4, the larger the shift on the position is, the larger the error. By displacing the RFA probe around 7 mm from its actual position, the mean error in the recovered thermal map is only 4.0 °C. This simulation analysis suggests robustness of the proposed method to the presence of errors in the RFA probe localization.

3.3 *Ex vivo* Feasibility Study

Two *ex vivo* experiments were performed on two chicken breast tissue samples. A PZT element was inserted 2.4 cm away from the RFA probe and a 6 cm linear probe of 128 elements (UltraSonix L14-5W/60) was used. To ensure a good in-plane alignment, the PZT element position was adjusted until we observed the

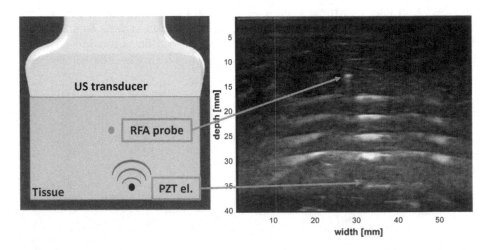

Fig. 5. (Left) Experimental setup: the US imaging probe is placed on top of the tissue. (Right) B-mode image acquired during the ablation: the RFA probe, the active PZT element and the virtual PI (four distant lines) are visible.

highest contrast in the B-mode image. The active element transmits four pulse trains with designed delay after detecting a line trigger from the US machine [3]. The ablation protocol used was as follows: heating was applied for 10–13 min followed by a 5-minute cooling period. We collected sequential B-mode images with PI during the ablation. The RFA probe and inserted PZT element positions were obtained from a pre-operative B-mode image, as illustrated in Fig. 5. Visual observation of the B-mode image during ablation showed changes in intensity and positions of the patterns over time. These variations were similar to those observed in the simulated B-mode images. Although no thermal ground truth was available for those *ex vivo* experiments, these qualitative observations suggest the suitability of the proposed concept Fig. 5, right.

4   Discussion and Conclusion

In this paper, a new paradigm for the interventional monitoring of temperature during thermal ablation is presented. The proposed method uses an active ultrasound (US) pattern injection (PI) system and relies on a learning tool based on a biophysical model of thermal ablation coupled with the simulation of B-mode images with PI. US is the imaging modality commonly used to guide the RFA probe insertion. Moreover, the method does not require to have access to the raw RF data from the US transducer (so-called channel or pre-beamformed RF data) only available on specialized US research platforms. For those reasons, this method might have a broad impact on the clinical practice. If available in real-time, the provided information could be used as feedback to adapt treatment parameters such as heating duration and/or power.

This work is a proof of concept with highly idealistic simulation and preliminary *ex vivo* results to show that biophysical modeling can be combined with virtual PI to monitor the temperature intraoperatively. To validate this novel concept, we chose a simplistic learning tool with a basic 2D cross-correlation metric to compare its elements to the acquired B-mode image. However, any learning tool could be considered. For example, a machine learning approach could be used to improve the applicability scope of the method by taking into account different settings (RFA probe positions, different heating protocols, etc.).

A major limitation of this work is its tissue parameter dependency. We assumed SoS and attenuation temperature dependencies from functions previously derived on different tissues [7,8]. While these assumptions were deemed satisfactory to assess the method feasibility, further investigations are required to evaluate their impact on the accuracy. The biophysical model could also consider the blood perfusion, heterogeneous tissue, as well as patient-specific parameters [1]. The effect of limited knowledge about those parameters was not evaluated but is important to consider in the future.

Nevertheless, we have showed that the current method is able to cope with noise in the raw RF data amplitude and motion on the image features used for temperature estimation. Furthermore, we have proposed an implementation for *ex vivo* experiments that warrants the validation with a thermal ground truth.

In conclusion, our results showed the method feasibility *in silico*. Future work will investigate quantitative evaluation using *in vivo* experiment settings.

Acknowledgments. Research reported in this paper was supported by the National Institute of Biomedical Imaging and Bioengineering of the National Institutes of Health under award number R01EB021396.

References

1. Audigier, C., Mansi, T., Delingette, H., Rapaka, S., Mihalef, V., Carnegie, D., Boctor, E., Choti, M., Kamen, A., Ayache, N., Comaniciu, D.: Efficient lattice Boltzmann solver for patient-specific radiofrequency ablation of hepatic tumors. IEEE Trans. Med. Imaging **34**(7), 1576–1589 (2015)
2. de Senneville, B.D., Mougenot, C., Quesson, B., Dragonu, I., Grenier, N., Moonen, C.T.W.: MR thermometry for monitoring tumor ablation. Eur. Radiol. **17**(9), 2401–2410 (2007)
3. Guo, X., Kang, H.-J., Etienne-Cummings, R., Boctor, E.M.: Active ultrasound pattern injection system (AUSPIS) for interventional tool guidance. PLoS ONE **9**(10), e104262 (2014)
4. Kim, Y., Guo, X., Boctor, E.M.: New platform for evaluating ultrasound-guided interventional technologies. In: Proceedings of SPIE, vol. 9790 (2016)
5. Lewis, M.A., Staruch, R.M., Chopra, R.: Thermometry and ablation monitoring with ultrasound. Int. J. Hyperth. **31**(2), 163–181 (2015)
6. Pennes, H.H.: Analysis of tissue and arterial blood temperatures in the resting human forearm. J. Appl. Physiol. **85**(1), 5–34 (1998)
7. Sun, Z., Ying, H.: A multi-gate time-of-flight technique for estimation of temperature distribution in heated tissue: theory and computer simulation. Ultrasonics **37**(2), 107–122 (1999)
8. Techavipoo, U., Varghese, T., Chen, Q., Stiles, T.A., Zagzebski, J.A., Frank, G.R.: Temperature dependence of ultrasonic propagation speed and attenuation in excised canine liver tissue measured using transmitted and reflected pulses. J. Acoust. Soc. Am. **115**(6), 2859–2865 (2004)
9. Tempany, C.M.C., Stewart, E.A., McDannold, N., Quade, B.J., Jolesz, F.A., Hynynen, K.: MRI-guided focused ultrasound surgery of uterine leiomyomas: a feasibility study 1. Radiology **226**(3), 897–905 (2003)
10. Treeby, B.E., Jaros, J., Rendell, A.P., Cox, B.T.: Modeling nonlinear ultrasound propagation in heterogeneous media with power law absorption using a k-space pseudospectral method. J. Acoust. Soc. Am. **131**(6), 4324–4336 (2012)

Erratum to: A Novel Ultrasound Imaging Method for 2D Temperature Monitoring of Thermal Ablation

Chloé Audigier[1,2(✉)], Younsu Kim[1], and Emad Boctor[1,2]

[1] Department of Computer Science, Johns Hopkins University,
Baltimore, MD, USA
caudigil@jhmi.edu
[2] Department of Radiology, Johns Hopkins University, Baltimore, MD, USA

Erratum to:
Chapter "A Novel Ultrasound Imaging Method for 2D Temperature Monitoring of Thermal Ablation"
in: M.J. Cardoso et al. (Eds.): Imaging for Patient-Customized Simulations and Systems for Point-of-Care Ultrasound, LNCS 10549, https://doi.org/10.1007/978-3-319-67552-7_19

The original version of the paper starting on p. 154 was revised. An acknowledgment has been added on p. 162. The original chapter has been corrected.

The updated online version of this chapter can be found at
https://doi.org/10.1007/978-3-319-67552-7_19

© Springer International Publishing AG 2017
M.J. Cardoso et al. (Eds.): BIVPCS/POCUS 2017, LNCS 10549, p. E1, 2017.
https://doi.org/10.1007/978-3-319-67552-7_20

Author Index